Praise for Matthew Pryor a

"In *The Body Tithe Devotional*, Matthew Pryor weaves inspiration and information to drive anyone with a body and soul to change. Matthew's transparency, insightful tips and godly direction inspired me to take action."

Kyle Idleman
Best-Selling Author of *Not a Fan*

"Every person who uses *The Body Tithe Devotional* will grow and mature in their knowledge and understanding of living the Christian life. This will serve to both inspire and instruct the reader to be a happy, healthy person in Christ. I give it a '10' for content, Scripture application, and ease in understanding."

Josh McDowell
Best-Selling Author of *More Than A Carpenter*

"I greet each New Year resolved to get in better physical condition! Do you? Unfortunately, our resolutions don't lead to slim, physically fit bodies because we lack a plan to keep our commitment. In *The Body Tithe Devotional*, Matthew Pryor shares his realistic plan to improve our spiritual and physical fitness. Buy his book. Apply it to your life. You'll be amazed at your new walk with Christ."

Bob Russell
Author of *Acts of God*

"For Pryor, fitness is not just a health issue, but a heart issue: Christians should be good stewards of physical health because our bodies are temples of the Holy Spirit (1 Corinthians 6:19) . . . Pryor shares about his own weight struggles as a child, but convincingly shows that fitness victory is not about a number on the scale. It's about honoring God with our bodies."

***World* Magazine**

"Matthew has knocked it out of the park with this devotional. He seamlessly integrates a believer's physical, mental and spiritual aspects into the whole person—this is a true 'Total Athlete' devotional! . . . This is a must read for the believer who wants to go deeper in their spiritual life, but stay connected to the importance of their fitness journey. Thanks Matthew!"

Mark Householder
President of Athletes in Action

"I love the concept of *The Body Tithe*! This 90-day journey is a life changer. Daily motivation to become who God truly called us to be—both physically and spiritually. Plan for a victory in Christ!"

Dave Stone
Pastor of Southeast Christian Church in Louisville, KY

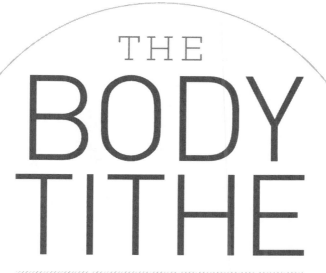

THE BODY TITHE

DEVOTIONAL

*Spiritual Encouragement for
Your Fitness Journey*

MATTHEW PRYOR

Printed in the United States of America
First Printing, 2015

ISBN 978-0-9970385-0-7

Sophros, LLC
9700 Park Plaza Avenue
Suite 203
Louisville, KY 40241

www.bodytithe.com

TABLE OF CONTENTS

ACKNOWLEDGMENTS

In no particular order, I want to thank those who have helped make this book possible:

My editor, Robert Sutherland. Thank you for your encouraging words and for challenging me to be a better writer than I wanted to be. I was ready to settle and you wouldn't let me. I thank you, as do the readers of this book.

My brothers in Christ, Rick Kelley and Ronnie Cordrey. Your faithful prayers over the course of this project served as a constant comfort.

Mexican food.

My longtime friend and mentor, Barney Long. Thank you for pouring into me all those years ago. Your words still echo in my ears and give me confidence to pursue whatever the Lord puts in front of me.

My brothers Andrew and Tre and your families. Your love and support throughout my life have been a priceless resource I have come to rely on time and time again.

My parents, Austin and Susie. It's cliché to say that I have the best parents in the world. So instead I'll say, I have the perfect parents for me. Your wisdom, love, and prayers have never been absent or in doubt. Thank you for modeling a godly marriage and for being obedient to the Lord's plans for your lives.

Gertie, my canine shadow. Your wordless support spoke volumes.

My children—Jordan, Myla, Gigi, and Silas. I wish you could comprehend the depths of my love for you. Someday, when you have children of your own, you'll understand. Until then just know that your crazy Daddy is crazy in love with you.

Phil Wickham and your music. John MacArthur and your writing. Neither man have I met, but your talents were a continual source of inspiration and insight throughout the composition of this book.

Thank you, church cookies. More specifically, to whoever came up with the recipes. Seriously, they're amazing.

Finally, my wife Kim. Thank you for believing in me. Thank you even more so for saying "I do" on that perfect October day in 1999. You are a role model, a blessing, and a delight to all those around you, including me. I don't deserve you.

'm the youngest of three sons, separated by roughly four and eight years from my brothers. I was active and healthy when I was young, but I was chubby. You probably wouldn't have thought twice about it, as I didn't stand out in a crowd. I stood out in my own eyes, though. No matter how charming I was (and trust me, I was plenty charming), at some point the chubby got the focus.

I'm 41 now, but I still remember an episode in third grade or so. I was sitting on the stairs in the basement of one of my best friends. We must have been roughhousing and sweaty because I didn't have my shirt on. When he saw my fat rolls, he pointed at them and commented. I don't even think he was being malicious . . . it just came out. Nevertheless, thirty-some-odd years later, I can still feel that remark.

One summer break in middle school, some friends (who were girls) sent me a postcard from Florida. On the front of it was some ripped dude in Speedos. On the back they wrote, "You wish." They were trying to be funny, but they weren't very good at it (and my mom certainly didn't like it either).

Another time in middle school, I remember playing dodgeball during recess. Must have been one of my less charming days because I got into a little bit of a shouting match. A kid on the other team yelled, "Well, at least I'm not chubby." I even remember where I was in the gymnasium when he said it. That was thirty years ago.

I remember in high school not wanting to take my shirt off at swim parties or for shirts/skins basketball games. On the basketball team, I was a decent shooter. I didn't get much playing time, though, in part because I was so slow. I was one of the last to finish any kind of speed drill. I dreaded practice because of the running and the humiliation. That was twenty-five years ago.

It wasn't until my early twenties that I got in really good shape for the first time. It felt awesome. There was no going completely back to the old me. That said, there certainly would be "lulls." During one such lull on family vacation, someone said to me, "Remember when you used to be in really good shape?" I know my family loves me and wants the best for me, and it probably just slipped out. But it hurt. That was probably 13 years ago. I don't think I've had much of a lull since then.

If it doesn't kill you, it just makes you stronger, right? Well, in this case, yes. It was a legitimate source of motivation for me. At the time, I certainly wouldn't have been thankful for the statements people made. They created insecurities and wounded feelings. Now that I've healed, though, I'm grateful, as they serve to propel me. There are scars but no pain. Only reminders of where I was and where I wanted to be.

God also was doing a work in me. I believe He allowed me to go through those trials for a reason. That reason became clearer as I matured more and more in my faith.

Romans is an incredible book in the Bible, layered with insights and revelations that build and encourage one's faith. Chapter eight in particular always leaves me feeling upbeat, especially when you read verses like this:

> *"And we know that in all things God works for the good of those who love him, who have been called according to his purpose."*
> *—verse 28 (NIV)*

For me, the work He was doing opened my eyes to the importance of fitness. He invigorated me to dig deeper into the relationship my fitness had to my faith. In turn, my motivation for my fitness changed.

Yes, I still look to achieve certain physical results. However, my overall goal is singular in purpose: to honor God with my body.

The mind, body, and spirit relationship can be a difficult one to understand. Certainly they're entwined, but to what extent? It's hard to know for certain. We know from Genesis that the body came first, and then life was breathed into it. In fact, the KJV reads not just "life" but "soul." Genesis 2:7 reads, "And the LORD God formed man of the dust of the ground, and breathed into his nostrils the breath of life; and man became a living soul." The breath of God is what makes us us. Our bodies seem to merely hold the true us.

C. S. Lewis would likely agree. He is often accredited with saying, "You don't have a soul. You are a soul. You have a body." I tend to side with this viewpoint. We are not given new souls when we enter into heaven; we are given new bodies (Philippians 3:21). If we are a body, how would we be given new bodies in heaven?

Nevertheless, as we learn more about the human body, we learn just how closely it is related to our emotions. For instance, our thought life can have a profound effect on the physiology of our brain. There are neural pathways in your brain that can be physically altered based on the things you're processing. Thinking about food can make you salivate and release digestive enzymes, hormones, and acids in your stomach. Both are physical responses to emotional stimuli.

Of course, what affects our soul can easily affect our body and vice versa. Ever been deeply grieving and felt either famished or overly satiated? Or perhaps experiencing seasons of especially intense joy has led you to feel huge surges of energy. Or maybe when you periodically experience the truth of His grace in your life. It hits you in an especially deep, penetrating level and you are moved to tears of gratitude. Or sorrow. Or both. All are physical reactions to spiritual occurrences. Whether we have a body or are part-body isn't the issue we are tackling. We are concerned with what we do with our bodies and why.

Ephesians 6:12 says, "For our struggle is not against flesh and blood, but against the rulers, against the authorities, against the powers of this dark world and against the spiritual forces of evil in the heavenly realms." In some ways, this can muddy the waters. It can give us license to ignore the proper caretaking of our bodies, since it's a "spirit" issue anyway. Like when I'm craving several slices of meat-lovers pizza for breakfast. Or when I'm considering sleeping in again rather than working out. My body wants what my body wants and I should give in. Besides, if I look, feel or act unhealthy, well, it doesn't really matter. Man looks at the outward appearance but God looks at the heart (wink-wink), right (wink-wink)?

Or equally bad, Ephesians 6:12 can have us over-spiritualizing everything. *Donuts aren't healthy. Satan doesn't want me to be healthy. So I should never eat a donut . . . or meat-lovers pizza . . . or sleep in.* Pretty soon we're ascribing morality to things of a neutral nature. This leads to us missing out on things God has given us for our enjoyment. Or even worse, we end up adopting a "works" mentality, performing for our approval rather than living out our approval.

On the flipside, this verse gives us much comfort. If we are spirit beings first, by default we are physical beings second. That means our battles are spiritual battles that manifest themselves at times physically. Yet we have access to the one who has *already* won the battles. If the victory is already His, then we don't do this on our own. He does it for us. We don't rely on our own strength for *any* of it; we rely on His strength for *all* of it.

This should bring us tremendous comfort. It means that this is first a spiritual issue. It means that honoring God with our bodies begins by honoring God with our hearts. To honor God only with our bodies does not really honor Him at all.

Read Matthew 23 and you'll see that Jesus is not a big fan of hypocrisy. What flows naturally out of honoring God in our hearts should be a compulsion to honor Him with our bodies. A desire to bring Him glory in *all* areas of our lives. While this book deals with fitness specifically, because it is a heart issue, the principles are universal. They can be applied to the stewardship of our time, money, gifts, family, jobs, influence, and so on. We are merely stewards. We are, however, His stewards. Therefore, we should be excited that He has chosen us to bring Him glory.

Okay, so how do we do that? How do we honor God with our hearts first? We seek to be fully and only satisfied by Him. You see, the more we are satisfied in Him, the harder it is to be satisfied with anything else. Not food. Not sleep. Not endorphins. Not a fitness-model physique or Samson-like strength. Not a sub-three-hour marathon. Not the compliments of friends. Not a glowing annual check-up. Definitely not the mirror.

Here's the extra cool part. The more we are satisfied in Him, the freer we become. We are freer to enjoy the benefits that come with living a healthier lifestyle. Imagine that! Living a life pleasing to the Lord benefits us. What an amazing design God has for our lives.

My prayer for you for the next 90 days is that you get a glimpse. A glimpse of just how big our God is. A glimpse of how very capable He is to orchestrate all things for His glory. A glimpse of who is with you in the battles of life. A glimpse of a victory that is already won.

A glimpse is all we need. Out of it we have hope. Great hope. For then we see that being completely nourished spiritually compels us to glorify Him physically.

Not out of guilt, but out of gratitude.

Not forcefully, but freely.

Not in tears, but in triumph!

HOW TO USE THIS BOOK

The first thing you should know is that every journey has phases, including a fitness journey. This is especially true for someone who is new to fitness. These phases are part physical, based on the strength you are gaining or stamina that's increasing, weight that you are losing, or _____.

You have to be *very* careful, though. If you let these results dictate your motivation, you can quickly go to an ugly place emotionally. You have to be on guard. Emotionally there are going to be many ups and downs throughout the 90 days. The goal is to maximize the ups and minimize the downs.

You see, fitness is as much emotional as it is physical, if not more. Again, we can't let the physical results decide for us how we will behave. Neither can we let what we experience emotionally be in charge. That's why it's essential as Christians to first approach our fitness from a spiritual point of view. By allowing God to align our wills to His, the spiritual can power both the physical and emotional.

The phases and their timelines are not identical for everyone, but they're certainly very close for most. By my estimate, there are six such phases. Therefore, as you go through this journey, know that phases are coming. When you are aware of them ahead of time, you will be better equipped to handle them. Below is a summary of each phase:

Weeks 1–3: Fire Phase
You're on fire! Excited to get started. Excited about the new exercise routine and even the nutrition. Excited because you see some physical changes.

Weeks 4–6: Flame Phase
You're still warm, but not nearly as hot as you were in the first phase. Early results start to taper and the realization that this is a lifestyle starts to set in. While you're still interested in the pursuit, the fire has certainly faded to a flame.

Week 7: Fizzle Phase

Your results have plateaued, which drives you in the wrong direction emotionally. Add to this that the novelty of newness is completely gone and the flame is now barely an ember. **This is the danger zone, where most people fall off the wagon.**

Weeks 8–10: Fortitude Phase

Okay, at this point you're just over it. Bad nutrition, missed workouts, and poor sleep are becoming more regular. To compound matters, your frustration makes you less inclined to make the right decisions, not more inclined. This is when it's essential just to keep showing up day after day. Like hitting "the wall" in a marathon, you have to just keep putting one foot in front of the next. **If you do that, some new results start emerging again toward the end of this phase.**

Week 11: Flare Phase

Your persistence in the previous phase is paying off! You're seeing some new results start to emerge. Furthermore, you're getting into a routine, learning better nutrition, improving your sleep, and nearing the end of the journey. There's light at the end of the tunnel. The feeling of satisfaction and pride gives you a confidence that starts to reignite the fire.

Weeks 12–13: Fun Phase

You're realizing the fruits of your labor. **You're learning that hard work works!** Fitness as a lifestyle is now realistic for you, and you're elated that you didn't give up. Your enthusiasm is not only contagious, but you find yourself helping others with their fitness.

Again, these phases aren't identical for everyone, but they hold generally true for most people. By getting ahead of them and expecting them to come, you'll be better equipped for the coming 90 days.

There are many reasons this book is based on a 90-day timeline. First, I think it takes at least that long to build lasting habits, despite what others may say. The longer you consistently do something, the better the chance it sticks.

Also, there are a number of great 90-day workout programs you can do at home. For those programs that are shorter, you can combine them with other programs. Or you can do multiple rounds of the same program. Whatever you decide to do workout-wise, *do not* try to shorten the duration. Commit to the full 90 days of your workouts, your eating program and the material you read in the devotional. Pray that God would teach you whatever He would like to teach you throughout these three months.

Second, BodyTithe.com offers challenge groups for its members. It's a safe place for members to be held accountable in a loving, gracious way. Members are encouraged to ask questions, share their struggles and their victories, and build community as together, they learn what Biblical body stewardship looks like. This is the only place where officially sanctioned groups are administered. Members of BodyTithe.com also have access to all the other content and tools on the site, each designed to help them develop a God-focused fitness mindset.

"We also created *The Body Tithe Devotional Study Guide* for those who want to go into greater depth with the material. Through daily journaling, challenging questions, heart-changing reflection, fitness tips, scripture writing and more, *The Body Tithe Devotional Study Guide* equips you to draw into an even stronger relationship with your Heavenly Father. The guide will help you apply scripture to your fitness, grow in your reliance on the Holy Spirit, find the root of your fitness struggles, and form an action plan for victory. A "Leader's Guide" is also included for those who want to lead a local small group, church class, or their own online group.

While *The Body Tithe Devotional Study Guide* is optional, we believe it is an excellent adjunct to the devotional itself, helping you to strengthen your prayer life, your walk with Christ, and your physical fitness."

Next, remember, all this material was designed to be used alongside other wellness programs in which you might be participating: group fitness classes, Weight Watchers, at home DVD programs, running groups, CrossFit, church small groups and Bible studies, your neighborhood walking groups, strength training with a buddy at the Y, and so on. The more accountability the better. As a group, it is easy to weave the lessons into your current fitness regimen.

Since accountability is so important, we also have a resource for those who are not members of BodyTithe.com. We created a *free* "Leader's Guide" to help those interested in leading others through this 13-week journey. If you're intimidated by being a "leader," don't be. We have created daily posts you can cut and paste straight into your group. These groups can be administered through Facebook, email, face-to-face, message board forums, or even in text messages. We even created some images you can use to keep people encouraged and motivated. Being a leader simply takes a servant's heart and a little vulnerability. The payoff of having God use you to guide others through this material is priceless. To download the free Leader's Guide, visit www.bodytithe.com/leadersguide.

Speaking of this material, some clarifications need to be made from the start. This is how I've defined fitness:

Fitness = Nutrition + Exercise + Sleep

Nutrition, exercise, and sleep are not equal, but the sum of their parts will help determine your overall fitness level. So when you read the word "fitness" you need to be thinking, "exercise, nutrition, and sleep."

You will also notice that each week you will have a new "Daily Spiritual Exercise." This exercise is to be practiced every day, throughout the day, for that week. You'll have 13 of these exercises, each one practiced for seven days. *Please do not skip these exercises.*

They are each designed to reinforce what you're learning that week and to keep you focused on the right things. Plus, they help keep the material you're learning relevant throughout the day. Five minutes a day is not enough. We want to be mindful of it all day. We are building spiritual muscles here! Again, don't short-change yourself or this process by skipping them. If you don't think you can make them a priority now, save the book for a time when you can.

Each day, you will also have a "Prayer" and a "Meditation." They are prayers I felt led to pray after having written the material. If you feel led to pray in a different direction, so be it. I would encourage you, however, to keep the listed meditation for each day. The meditation stems from that day's reading and corresponds with the app.

Finally, I talk about this journey in the context of 90 days. Obviously, our fitness (for good or bad) doesn't stop after that. It's lifelong. My prayer then is that you'll spend your life pursuing His heart. As you do, He will help you work out your fitness with fear and trembling.

WEEK 1 PREVIEW
Names for Jesus

We play a great game around our dinner table. It's called the "What do you like about?" game. We go around the table, saying things we like about a family member. It's especially gratifying to hear what the kids say: "Mommy is kind." "Daddy is silly." "Mommy is a hard worker." Or one of my personal faves: "Daddy is a beast." While we can never put into words how much our family means to us, it sure is fun to try.

When you think of some of the most respected Christians of all time, how would you describe them? John the Baptist. Mother Teresa. Jim Elliot. Bill Bright. The Apostle Paul. C. S. Lewis. Billy Graham. Peter. We are in awe of people like this and rightfully so. They were fiercely obedient to the call God placed on their hearts, costing some of them their lives. If we played the "What do you like about?" game, we could easily come up with four or five attributes that could sum up the depth of their character.

When we think of Jesus, though, the greatest man of all time, summarizing suddenly gets harder. There just are not enough words in all the languages on Earth. No human descriptions could adequately capture the profundity of who He was and is. But it sure is fun to try.

To get the fun started, we need to look no further than Scripture. Some of the most poignant, descriptive, and apt titles for the only man to have lived perfectly reside there. The only man on whom calendars are founded. The only man to have conquered death. The only man who has the authority to give eternal life.

The more we understand who He is, the better we can rely on Him. The better we rely on Him for our everything, the more we can understand Him. Then we realize that the names attributed to Jesus equip us! They equip us to deal with our jobs, focus on our families, face our trials, and handle our health. All the names of Jesus equip us to bring glory back to God and experience victory . . . daily.

Yet, as each name flawlessly portrays the person of Christ, each one is also inadequate on its own—helpful but still only pieces of a much bigger puzzle. Start connecting the pieces, however, and an image appears. A beautiful, overwhelming, and life-shattering glimpse of Christ emerges. However, on this side of heaven, it will only ever be a glimpse. There just aren't enough pieces to complete the puzzle.

But it sure is fun to try.

Daily Spiritual Exercise: Pray without ceasing.
While Jesus was fully God, he was also fully man. He remained sinless because He remained in constant communion with the Father. If the Son of Man needed to be in constant communion with God, how much more do we need it?

We need it in every area of our lives, fitness included. Fitness is a struggle for many, but nothing is a struggle for God. He wants to help you with it and He is more than able. In order for Him to help, though, He needs to be the one to do it on our behalf. He needs to be the one to power it.

Set a reminder on your watch, phone or computer to go off every hour (or even more frequently). This is a reminder to pray, to stay in constant connection with God, to realign your mind, will, and purposes to His. You don't have to stop and drop to your knees (though you can if you'd like). Just converse with Him in your heart and mind. Surrender your will to His and ask for His strength to help you during this fitness journey. We are seeking a permanently open dialogue with God. Do this every day this week and pray that He helps you make it second nature.

Remember: the more we remain in Him, the more victory we will experience in all areas of our lives.

Week 1 Day 1 | *Names for Jesus: Cornerstone*

Have you ever seen a cornerstone on a historical building? Maybe you've even seen one decorated with a relief or inscription of some kind. These are pretty much ceremonial these days, but in earlier times they had a purpose beyond decoration.

The cornerstone was the first stone set in construction of a foundation requiring masonry. Notice it was not only part of the foundation, but it was the first part of the foundation. Since it came before anything else, all the other stones would have been set in reference to it. An imperfect or misplaced cornerstone would alter the position and integrity of the entire structure.

However, using a cornerstone that's true changes everything. One with perfect 90-degree right angles. A building block that has straight edges and level base. Construct your foundation out from there and you'll have a building that can last . . . that can stand the test of time.

Understanding the purpose of a cornerstone in biblical times provides context for the significance of this description given to Jesus:

> *"Together, we are his house, built on the foundation of the apostles and the prophets. And the cornerstone is Christ Jesus himself."—Ephesians 2:20 (NLT)*

Jesus certainly needs to be the cornerstone of the church and of our faith. He also needs to be the cornerstone of our goals, motives and intentions, decisions, and ambitions. Since He's the only perfect cornerstone, all other cornerstones by definition are off. They will result in misaligned ambitions, unstable decisions, wobbly motives, and shaky goals that, over time, will crumble. Other cornerstones will always require us to rebuild.

We see this all the time with money, influence or jobs, and certainly with fitness. If the cornerstone of my fitness goals is to impress others, what happens when I fail to get feedback? What if I see someone else who is far more impressive than I am? My focus will become even more self-centered than it already was. If the cornerstone of my fitness is to look better, what happens when I stop seeing results in the mirror? Or if the results I see are never enough? I get discouraged, frustrated, and discontent. From there, I'm likely to compromise my nutrition, exercise or sleep. Nor should "Feeling better" be the cornerstone of our fitness. What happens if we never feel better, if we get hurt or diseased? Our attitude will quickly shift to one of apathy and laziness. When the focus is about us, the building we're erecting becomes less and less stable. It is unable to survive high winds or the weight of a heavy snow.

This is not to say that having fitness goals is wrong. In fact, I encourage them. They give us quantifiable data to shoot for, measure progress against and can teach us how to make adjustments. They can also reveal how we are wired. However, our goals can also unknowingly trick us. They become the purpose for our fitness. That's why goals and focus should never be synonymous. When our goals become our focus, Jesus is not. Before we know it, our goals have become our cornerstone.

However, with Jesus as the cornerstone of our fitness, He can lay the foundation. From that foundation, our reflection of Him might serve as a catalyst for others. Where looking better could be a result, rather than a point of focus. Where feeling better and performing better can be a natural byproduct of our efforts, rather than the emphasis of them.

It's essential to establish this from Day 1. Above all else, our goal should be to honor God with our fitness. We do this *not* by having Jesus merely involved. We do this by making Jesus the cornerstone. Then and only then will we have a foundation that is true. One that is sound, without cracks and unsusceptible to settling. One that is solid, impermeable to torrential downpours and flash floods. One that is strong, sturdy enough to withstand the emotional earthquakes that come with living in an imperfect world.

Sound. Solid. Strong. Certainly a description worthy of our Jesus.

Prayer

Father, thank You for your son Jesus, the perfect Cornerstone. Thank you that He wants to be at the basis of our lives, decisions, and motives. Will You forgive me when I let the primary focus of my fitness be anything other than Him? Please gently remind me to continually build my faith on Him, a foundation void of cracks, unmovable, and everlasting. Amen.

Meditation

Jesus, the Cornerstone of my faith, the foundation of my life.

Daily Spiritual Exercise

Pray without ceasing.

Week 1 Day 2 | *Names for Jesus: Bread of Life*

Outside of your genetics, there are three things that will determine your level of fitness: exercise, nutrition, and sleep. Nutrition is arguably the most important. Hippocrates said, "Let food be thy medicine, and medicine be thy food." For the physical body, there's a ton of truth to that. So it's important to focus on learning how to eat smart right from the get-go.

For Christians working on their health, however, I would argue that your spiritual nutrition trumps even your physical nutrition. Since we are early in this fitness journey, now is the time to learn how to feed our bodies spiritually. As you will see in the coming weeks, that's where most of the wars are waged.

There's no more fitting analogy for our spiritual nutrition than Jesus as the "Bread of Life." Now when I think of Jesus as the Bread of Life, it's almost always during Communion. I default to the Last Supper. My mind's eye sees Jesus breaking the bread and telling his disciples to eat it in remembrance of Him.

At our church, we have the great and humbling privilege of taking Communion every week. It's a time I dread and cherish simultaneously. As I'm holding the cup of juice and the piece of bread, I think back on my week. I always fall so short of living the kind of holy life we are called to live. While I know I'm forgiven and there's no condemnation, it's hard not to be a little embarrassed sitting there. I'm confessing the same sin that I've confessed countless times before, asking to be forgiven yet again. At the root of my sin, anyone's sin actually, is the simple failure to be nourished solely by Jesus. It's not all that complicated, really. I've gone away from someone who was given to fulfill and satisfy in favor of something that never will.

So why do I reserve the notion of Jesus as the Bread of Life for weekly Communion? I can ponder it all the time, everywhere, no matter what! Jesus certainly didn't confine it to Communion. In fact, He first referred to himself as the "Bread of Life" in John 6 after He had fed the five thousand, which was well before the Last Supper.

In His perfect timing, after first attending to the physical needs of the people, He focuses on their spiritual needs. He tells His disciples in verse 27: "Do not work for food that spoils, but for food that endures to eternal life, which the Son of Man will give you." Then He follows up a few verses later with:

> "Then Jesus declared, 'I am the bread of life. Whoever comes to me will never go hungry, and whoever believes in me will never be thirsty.'"—verse 35 (NIB)

What would happen if I consistently fed my spirit on the Bread of Life rather than settling for "food that spoils?" I will tell you what would happen, I would not go hungry!

Practically speaking, what does this look like in relationship to our fitness? For starters, it means being alert to the temptation to seek our fulfillment from other sources. When we're having a bad day and we reach for junk food to make us feel better, we're reaching for food that spoils. There's a better option: food that "gives life to the world," as Jesus stated in John 6:32. He is life, and His life can sustain us spiritually on earth and eternally in heaven.

How do we remain alert? By abiding in Him. By taking on the mind of Christ. By praying without ceasing, listening to His whispers, and responding in obedience.

This also means that we can trust Him to take care of us during the harder times. In John 6:37, Jesus says, "whoever comes to me I will never drive away." On days when we're not motivated to exercise, perhaps we first need to go to Jesus. We can lay our very real struggle into His very capable hands and watch Him work in us for His glory.

As you're working on your physical nutrition over the course of these 13 weeks, focus first on your spiritual nutrition. Do not reserve the Bread of Life for Sundays. Make it a daily mindset.

While weekly Communion is good, constant communing is better.

Prayer

Father, thank You for being a source of everlasting fulfillment and endless satisfaction. Will You forgive me when I seek foods that don't satisfy . . . rather than your Son who does? Please give me wisdom with my health. Even more importantly, help me grow spiritually as I seek to honor You with my body. Amen.

Meditation

Jesus, You are the Bread of Life.

Daily Spiritual Exercise

Pray without ceasing.

Week 1 Day 3 | *Names for Jesus: Radiance of God's Glory*

Grasping the concept of the Trinity is hard and rightfully so. Our human minds struggle to understand the basics of a pre-earth timelessness (Psalm 90:2) or a post-earth eternity (Psalm 93:1–5). Then try comprehending how Jesus was both fully God and fully human simultaneously. Once you've mastered that, factor in how the Holy Spirit fits into the picture.

That's one reason I love the following verse so much. Not only does it paint a beautiful picture, it breaks down the relationship for us, making it easier to understand:

> *"The Son is the radiance of God's glory and the exact representation of his being, sustaining all things by his powerful word."*
> —Hebrews 1:3 (NIV)

Radiance, or brightness, comes from the Greek word *apaugasma*, meaning "to send forth light." God's glory was manifested in Jesus, "the representation of his being." Jesus was sent forth, yet never separated from God the Father, as they are the same (John 4:9–11).

John MacArthur puts it like this: "Just as the sun was never without and cannot be separated from its brightness, so God was never without and cannot be separated from the glory of Christ. Never was God without Him or He without God, and never in any way can He be separated from God. Yet the brightness of the sun is not the sun. Neither is Christ God in that sense. He is fully and absolutely God, yet is a distinct Person."

That means, by Jesus we have the means to relish God's light, the light of the world.

Every now and then, people will pay me a compliment by saying that I inspire them with their fitness. While I appreciate the sentiment, I cringe a little on the inside. I see this all the time on social media: someone who wants to be an "inspiration" for others. Yuck.

Our goal as Christians is not to be an "inspiration" but to be a "reflection." When we seek to inspire, the focus is on what we do. When we seek to reflect, it's on what God does. Inspiration is secondary. It's a by-product, not the goal.

Like the moon, we have no light source of our own. On our own, we do no good thing. We have no good thing (Psalm 16:2). We are solely dependent on the sun as our source of light. However, when we seek to reflect the Son, Jesus in us, working through us, He lights the way for others. He illuminates the darkness. He shines into hearts and makes them glow.

As you go through this journey, you will make some significant strides. You will be diligent with your nutrition and exercise. You'll prioritize your sleep and be refreshed from your rest. You will get noticeably more fit. As you enjoy these benefits of a healthy life, you will also inadvertently inspire others. When they bring this to your attention, the challenge is to find a way to reflect this back to God.

After all, we can't do this without Him. Jesus was quick to point back to His Father (Mark 10:18). We too should be quick to point back to our Jesus, because as Hebrews 1:3 concludes, He is sustaining all things . . . us included. We can do no good thing apart from him.

We are the moon.

Prayer
Father, thank You for sending the Light, your Son, the radiance of your Glory, to earth to give us hope and a future. Will You forgive me when I seek to inspire rather than reflect? Please give me the integrity and honesty to keep You as the source of my strength. Amen.

Meditation
Jesus is the Radiance of God's glory.

Daily Spiritual Exercise
Pray without ceasing.

Week 1 Day 4 | *Names for Jesus: Rabbi*

When you hear the name "Jesus," what's the first thing that comes to mind?

I'd venture to guess most people think of "Lord," "Son," or "Savior." Certainly they are all apt titles, but they weren't the most popular during His life on earth. The title he received more than any other by far was "Rabbi," which means "teacher":

> *"He came to Jesus at night and said, 'Rabbi, we know that you are a teacher who has come from God.'"–John 3:2a (NIV)*

As a sign of respect, His apostles addressed him this way, which certainly was not uncommon for the day. However, fast-forward two thousand years and it still is applicable for us. After all, everywhere He went He taught in such a way that we're still learning from Him. However, while most teachers have certain strengths, Jesus had no weaknesses; He was equally powerful whether He was teaching by word, by deed, or by example.

First, when you study the words Rabbi used, you quickly come to realize that He was a master wordsmith. His words were chosen with purpose, structured to shed light, bring life, stir the conscious, and create change. They were relatable. For instance, when talking to fishermen, Rabbi said He'd make them fishers of men (Matthew 4:19). His words were thought-provoking, as when He says that He didn't come to be served, but to serve (Mark 10:45). His words were challenging, as when Rabbi tells the disciples to love their enemies and do good for them (Luke 6:35). Certainly the Rabbi's parables were profound. Some go on to brand the heart for generations untold, as with the parable of the prodigal son.

However, as they say, "talk is cheap." Rabbi's words would have been hollow had they not been supported by His deeds. Of course, this was not the case. In fact, His deeds magnified the truth of His words, and vice versa. Wherever He went, Rabbi had compassion. This compassion resulted in attending to the physical needs of the people by miracles of healing (Matthew 15:30), feeding (Matthew 15:32–38), and resurrections (John 11:43–44).

Rabbi's compassion also resulted in more teaching. For instance, we read in Mark 6:34, "When Jesus landed and saw a large crowd, he had compassion on them, because they were like sheep without a shepherd. So he began teaching them many things." Notice His compassion came first. It led Him to begin teaching (and eventually multiplying the fish and bread). Teaching was the deed that magnified the truth of Rabbi's compassion.

Rabbi spoke perfectly, acted perfectly and by doing, He set the perfect example for us to follow. Sometimes, His example was impactful not because of what He said or did. It was because of what He didn't say or do. For instance, when Mary joins Jesus at her brother's tomb, John 11:35 tells us that "Jesus wept." He didn't tell her everything was going to be okay, though it was. He didn't set out to fix the situation, though it got fixed. He chose to empathize with Mary first. In so doing, He demonstrates that He can commiserate with our every emotion even while He can mend every situation. Rabbi teaches us that sometimes our loved ones just need to be listened to and understood.

We also see this principle played out in John 8. A woman caught in adultery, sentenced to be stoned, was first brought to Jesus. Yet rather than doing the expected, Rabbi did nothing. Rabbi withheld condemnation. He teaches us the unproductive nature of judging others. We again learn from Rabbi by what He didn't do.

Then, in the most perfect of all teaching moments, by word, deed, and example, Rabbi took our place on the cross. Rather than ruling by might, He serves in grace. All in one single act, He educated us on benevolence, humility, love, and sacrifice.

Over the course of this journey, if we are open, listening, and malleable, we will not stop learning from Rabbi. There is no end to the wisdom that can be found in His words. Even today, His words and the words of His Father are alive and active (Hebrews 4:12). Even at this very moment we can be trained in righteousness. We can be equipped for every good work, thanks to the life of Rabbi (2 Timothy 3:15–17).

Change, however, only happens if we let it. Knowledge is only helpful if we apply it. True spiritual growth only occurs if we allow Rabbi's words to penetrate and let the Holy Spirit work within us. When we permit these principles to shape our lives, we pave the way for Him to shape our fitness.

Consider adding "Rabbi" to the list of names you'd give Jesus. After all, in the history of everything that has ever been, no teacher can impact your heart, mind, and will as Rabbi can.

Prayer
Father, thank You for giving us Rabbi, the perfect teacher. Will You forgive me when I don't listen to what He's trying to teach me? Please keep enlightening His words in my heart and mind. Give me a willing spirit to put them into practice. Amen.

Meditation
From your teaching, Rabbi, I can never stop learning.

Daily Spiritual Exercise
Pray without ceasing.

Week 1 Day 5 | *Names for Jesus: The Shepherd and the Lamb*

We have a wonderful little Chihuahua-pug mix we adopted from a rescue shelter in 2003. When we got her, there weren't many, ahem, "chugs" around. She has a thick yellow coat, stocky frame, and the infamous curly tail. Her face is composed of small, soft ears with big, brown eyes overlooking a short, brown snout. At about 30 pounds, she is bigger than a traditional pug, but she's still all raspy bark, no bite. Based on her look we imagined that if she could talk, she'd have a German accent. So, we named her "Gertie," short for Gertrude.

Gertie acclimated to our then-family of three in no time. She has also been a perfect big sister to the three children we've added since. Sweet, mostly obedient, fun and easy to take care of, she has been the perfect dog for us. While she loves everyone, she is especially drawn to me. I was the one to learn she was available at the animal shelter. I also happened to be the one to first go visit her and also the one to bring her home. On some level, it seems like Gertie knows that I saved her. Consequently, she parked her ultimate allegiance with me. She greets me when I come home. She obeys when I command. She comes when I call. When we get back from a vacation, I get the lion's share of the kisses. When I say her name, her little triangle ears perk. She knows my voice and I know her bark.

Jesus has a similar relationship with us. We see this demonstrated in John 10, when He uses the analogy of the Shepherd and the sheep:

> *"I am the good shepherd; I know my sheep and my sheep know me . . ."*
> *—verse 14 (NIV)*

Throughout that passage in John, Jesus talks about what a shepherd does for the sheep. He calls them, defends them, leads them and ultimately would die for them. It's the perfect analogy to use because sheep are helpless, desperate, and dumb. Compared to our Shepherd, so are we. We are the Gerties of the world, needing to be defended, rescued, adopted, and loved. We need help.

As Gertie has gotten up there in years, she too has needed more and more help. Cysts removed. Teeth extracted. Blood tests, kidney tests and a daily supplement regimen to prevent future issues. The days of her being an inexpensive pet are long over. That said, she's worth it. She is a part of our family. Honestly, there's not much I wouldn't do for her. However, I wouldn't die for her. As much as I love her, I wouldn't lay my life down for hers. That's where the similarities end between our pets and us, and us and our Shepherd . . . He would die for us. He did die for us:

> *". . . just as the Father knows me and I know the Father and I lay down my life for the sheep . . ."–John 10:15 (NIV)*

Jesus is not merely our Shepherd. In fact, before we ever read about the Good Shepherd, we see John refer to Him as a lamb. In John 1:29 we read, "The next day John saw Jesus coming toward him and said, 'Look, the Lamb of God, who takes away the sin of the world!'" John calls Him "Lamb of God" again six verses later.

You know what? It only makes sense. Who else could be two opposite entities at the same time: the Shepherd and the Lamb? Who else could fully express the qualities of contrary lives without diminishing the relevance of either of them? If He weren't the Shepherd and the Lamb, the contrast to sin and the sacrifice for it, why trust Him? Would He be worth putting our hope in if He had to be confined to one virtue at a time? Would He be worth putting our faith in for our earthly living, let alone our eternal salvation?

As with Gertie, we have been rescued, adopted, and loved. We can be cared for, looked out after, and given what we need. We can have a family and a Father.

Unlike Gertie's "father," however, ours has the ability to empower our lives for eternity, while energizing our lives on earth. God can fuel our fitness, shape our focus, and strengthen our resolve. He can sharpen our perspective with the assurance of what his Son Jesus has done and will do for us.

He is both the doctor and the medicine. The teacher and the lesson. The ransom and the reward. The sun and the shade. The artist and the art. The demand and the supply. The Giver and the Gift. He's everything we need and nothing we don't.

He is the Shepherd and He is the Lamb.

Prayer
Father, thank You for sending your Shepherd-Son to be the sacrificial Lamb. Will You forgive me when You call and I don't come? Please help me to follow You, because only You are worth following.

Meditation
You lead and I will follow.

Daily Spiritual Exercise
Pray without ceasing.

Week 1 Day 6 | *Names for Jesus: The Author*

When you look at the story of your life, what perspective do you take? I think the temptation for most people is to look at it with a top-down view. With a vague deference given to some of the obvious age breaks, your life probably gets grouped into sections like this: childhood, high school and college, single, married, children, and so on. At the risk of making you hungry, it's as if we're looking at a piece of lasagna only from the top. We see a long rectangle, with a beginning, middle, and end (maybe some red sauce on the sides too). It's one-dimensional.

What we should be doing is looking at the lasagna from the side. Our lives are stories on top of stories on top of stories, like repeating layers of sauce, noodles, meat, and cheese. Take just one day, just one forkful, and you'll see a cross-section of stories stacked on top of one another: stories of relationships with your spouse, children, friends, and loved ones. Stories of a long work transition you've been going through and of a home improvement project you've been tackling. Stories of the volunteer work you've been doing and stories of the time spent at T-ball. Stories of your Bible reading routine in the morning and of your downtime television habit at night. With each bite, the story continues.

Where there is a story, there is an author. The stories of our lives are no different. What should be different for Christians, however, is we should entrust the plot to a much better writer than ourselves. After all, it's only prudent to hand over the pen to the One who invented the medium.

We see this description in Acts 3, when Peter addressed the crowd who had just seen him heal a lame man. He reminded them that it wasn't Peter who healed the man. It was Jesus, "the author of life." That same author, Jesus, can also be the author of our life.

The Author of Life is also known as the Author of Salvation, as we see in the 1984 NIV translation of Hebrews 2:10: "In bringing many sons to glory, it was fitting that God, for whom and through whom everything exists, should make the author of their salvation perfect through suffering." Wow! Read this part again: "for whom and through whom everything exists…" That's why we are here. That's how we are here.

We are here by Him and through Him. It's by His Son's suffering that our salvation has been authored.

Then, later in Hebrews, we're once again implored to turn to Jesus:

> *"Let us fix our eyes on Jesus, the author and perfecter of our faith, who for the joy set before him endured the cross, scorning its shame, and sat down at the right hand of the throne of God."*
> *—Hebrews 12:2 (NIV)*

Jesus authored eternal life by authoring salvation. He will author and perfect our faith as well, until we are united with Him again someday. The "until" is the hard part. The "until" is where we live out our days. It's the "until" that requires patience and perseverance. The good news is they don't come by our own hand. As we see over and over, the challenge is to relinquish the compulsion to write our own story.

With this fitness journey, you are starting another story, adding another layer. There are likely threads of fitness endeavors throughout the cross-section of your life. Perhaps what makes this story different is you've decided you will no longer be the one holding the pen. That lack of control makes you nervous but excited. The faith required to loosen your grip only adds to the passion and exhilaration of the tale He wants to tell. A story of trial and triumph. Of narrow escapes and grand victories. Of a life lived with courage, peace, and power.

Furthermore, when we are not responsible for writing the plot, we actually have more freedom, not less. When we no longer shoulder the burden of worry, fear or anxiety, we're freer to enjoy the process of Him perfecting our faith. We have but one concern: obedience, which is why we fix our eyes on the Son.

So, drop the pen. Put down the paper. You've surrendered the right to write any more. It's time to acknowledge that there's someone better suited for the task. A skilled wordsmith. A master creator.

A life giver, salvation maker, faith shaper, and perfect author.

Prayer

Father, thank You for giving me life and having a purpose for it. Will You forgive me when I'm determined to write my own story? Please help me to remain faithful, fixed on your Son, following in faithful obedience. Amen.

Meditation

Your hand writes my story.

Daily Spiritual Exercise

Pray without ceasing.

Week 1 Day 7 | *Names for Jesus: Morning Star*

I don't know about you, but I am not a morning person. Doesn't matter how early I go to bed or the restfulness of my sleep. Getting up early is just not my thing. So, I'm stuck with the commotion of noisy children, work tasks, to-do lists, and workouts to jolt me out of bed.

I wish getting up early did agree with me. I think my days would go smoother if I eased into reality. Plus, evidence suggests the most pro-ductive people are those who do get up well before the sun rises. More than that, there is an almost magical peace about an early morning: the space between night and light, before the world wakes up and the stars go to sleep. With dew resting, dawn rising and nature harmonizing, early mornings invite an introspective solitude that's nourishing, even if for just a moment.

Perhaps that's why the names of Jesus that relate Him to the morning resonate with me. They depict an intangible yet experiential quality that I desire to characterize my days. Depending on your translation, Luke 1:78 refers to Jesus as "the Dawn from on high," "the dayspring," "the morning light," and "the rising sun." In Malachi 4:2, we read, "the Sun of Righteousness arise…" Then, in 2 Peter 1:19 and later in Revelation, perhaps the most appropriate and poetic of the bunch—"the morning star":

> *"I, Jesus, have sent my angel to give you this message for the churches. I am both the source of David and the heir to his throne. I am the bright morning star."—Revelation 22:16 (NLT)*

Some interesting notes about the morning star. For starters, it isn't ac-tually a star at all. It's Venus. Of course, Venus is a planet and therefore does not produce any light of its own. It reflects the light of the sun. It's so good at reflecting the sun that Venus can even be seen during some of the brightest days. It's called "the morning star" because it precedes the sun morning . . . after morning . . . after morning.

As we learn more about the Morning Star, we start seeing why it's such a fitting description for Jesus. First, life on earth preceded the fulfillment and establishment of the heavenly Kingdom. While He was the light of the world, Jesus reflected His Father, staying in perfect communion with Him. Jesus shined brighter than anyone before Him or since. Just as celestial bodies do, Jesus gives direction. He helps us set our bearings.

If our fitness is to be successful, both physically and spiritually, the Morning Star will need to be our compass. Fortunately for us, His example shines morning . . . after morning . . . after morning. Jesus models and provides the consistency we need to seek in our fitness. We can set our sights on Him as the focus and destination of the journey. Then we can rely on the wisdom from the Holy Spirit to figure out the mechanics of it.

In the beginning, this is often easier because of the newness of the journey. Yet the excitement shouldn't only be in the newness of the process, but rather in the process itself, that every morning we are given a new day with another opportunity to pursue God-honoring body stewardship.

In so doing, we will be given opportunities to shine in one of two ways. One, we can try to inspire others by our example and in so doing, take the credit for the progress. That, however, results in being a mere flicker in the dark.

The other option is give the glory back to God. We can give Him credit for what He has done for us, in us, and through us. Then, we reflect His light, rather than trying to produce any of our own. Then, we are like His Son. Then, we can shine with a true brilliance that never ends and never dims.

That brilliance allows us to experience the supernatural peace of Jesus, a peace that surpasses understanding. We can experience the Creator of night and light. We experience the One who spins the world awake and put the stars to sleep. We experience the One who drops the dew on the grass, breaks the dawn and orchestrates the rhythms of nature. We get to do this with the One who invites us into a loving relationship that completely nourishes the soul . . . for life. We can do this day . . . after day . . . after day . . . so that it characterizes our lives.

With entire days like that, who needs mornings?

Prayer

Father, thank You for sending your Son to be The Morning Star. Will You forgive me when I model my life on anything other than Him? Please help me to keep Him as the source of my efforts. Amen.

Meditation

The Morning Star is the focus and the foundation of my fitness.

Daily Spiritual Exercise

Pray without ceasing.

WEEK 2 PREVIEW

Old Testament Heroes

The 39 books of the Old Testament read like something out of a Hollywood script—full of wonder and mystery, good and evil. With scandal and intrigue, special effects and romance, there is much entertainment on a surface level.

However, when we dig deep into the hearts of the protagonists, much is revealed. When we see what made them who they were, we learn a lot and are encouraged in the process. These heroes of faith were, in some ways, like you and me. They had jobs and families, strengths and weaknesses, insecurities and temptations, and moments of triumph and stretches of utter failure. It's both the triumphs *and* the failures that are so comforting.

Perhaps the greatest leader in the Bible was Moses. He led the ungrateful Israelites for forty years in the desert, evaded the enemy and performed epic miracles. That said, Moses also questioned the Lord, struggled with absolute obedience, and battled frustration. In the end, it prevented him from entering the Promised Land.

It's easy to be motivated by the righteousness of Joseph's integrity. However, many believe that Joseph had to overcome pride and arrogance as a young man.

Having been called "a man after God's own heart," David was an admirable friend, a worshipful poet, and skilled king. He was also an adulterer and a murderer.

We are blown away by Solomon. The Lord offers him anything, and Solomon asks for wisdom rather than wealth or a long life. In spite of that, Solomon was a weak man. He failed to rely on the strength of that very same wisdom. Solomon struggled with finding fulfillment and satisfaction in the Lord alone. As a result, he sought the love and company of thousands of wives and concubines.

Do you struggle with questions, insecurities, doubt, frustration, fulfillment, obedience, envy, pride, arrogance, or _____?

Me too! That's exactly why these stories are so encouraging. God led men and women into greatness in spite of their sin, the same sin we struggle with today. Our God delights in bringing good out of bad. God is a master at creating heroes out of the unremarkable, and making beauty spring from where none exists. All to bring glory back to His name.

So be encouraged! Heroes of the Bible were human just like us. What makes them heroes is how they allowed God to work through them. We can do the same thing!

Daily Spiritual Exercise: Meditate on an attribute of God.

Every day this week, you are going to meditate on an attribute of God, an attribute of your choosing. To get you started however, read Job chapters 38–41. (We will be taking a look at Job later this week.)

Sometimes in our humanity, we forget exactly who God is and we put limits on Him where there are none. This passage from Job quickly reminds us that nothing is beyond our God's abilities.

Week 2 Day 1 | *Old Testament Heroes: David*

King David occupies a fair amount of real estate in the Old Testament. His story is told in 1 Samuel, 2 Samuel, 1 Kings, and 1 Chronicles. David is mentioned in other books as well and is responsible for writing roughly half of the Book of Psalms. It is through David's lineage that Jesus comes to Earth.

When you think of David, what words come to mind? Brave . . . adulterer . . . poet . . . man after God's own heart . . . murderer? David really runs the full spectrum.

Today, we're going to look at one of the most famous of all stories in Scripture: David and Goliath. We will see from a couple of subtle but key references just how "intentional" David was at times.

We skip past Goliath's taunting and the wimpy, faithless Israelites cowering. We skip forward to the part where David volunteers to take on the behemoth. He foregoes the armor that was too big or heavy. He chooses instead what he finds most comfortable: his own skin and his own staff. So we read:

> *"Then he took his staff in his hand, chose five smooth stones from the stream, put them in the pouch of his shepherd's bag and, with his sling in his hand, approached the Philistine."—1 Samuel 17:40 (NIV)*

Now look again closely at verse 40 and the phrase, "chose five smooth stones from the stream." A few things might jump out.

First is the word "chose." *The Message* uses the word "selected." It implies that David didn't randomly grab or merely scoop up some rocks, but he was deliberate. We see this also by evidence of the fact that no ordinary stones would do. They needed to be "smooth." Why? Better aerodynamics? I don't know, but he knew what he wanted . . . no rough or chunky stones for David. David was intentional.

What's also interesting is that David chose five stones, not just one. David was a young man, full of faith. He was confident in the abilities of His God to dispose of the giant. Why then did David take five, when just one would do the trick? Did it show some doubt, some second-guessing or a lack of belief?

Not likely. If that were the case, why not choose 20 or 30 rocks? David was just being prepared. He was an experienced marksman who had killed lions and bears as he defended his father's sheep (1 Samuel 17:34–36). He had a history of taking down attackers. David understood that Goliath, at nearly 10 feet tall, might need more than one shot to take down. But it wasn't gonna take more than five! Again, David was intentional.

Ever heard the popular phrase, "Fail to plan and plan to fail"? How true that is in life, be it our spiritual life, family life, work life, and certainly our fitness life. After all, getting in shape doesn't just happen . . . we don't fall into shape. We fall out of shape.

One of the dirty little secrets about fitness is that 90 percent of the work comes outside of the gym. The real work comes in the sacrifice, the learning, the consistency, and most often in the planning. When we wing it, we botch it. We have to give our fitness forethought if it's going to become a part of our lifestyle. It takes planning, and planning is work. The better we get at planning, the easier it becomes.

However, planning is only part of the equation. You can succeed at planning, but still fail at execution if you're not intentional. David was an excellent marksman, having executed his skill a number of times. It was this combination of his planning, execution, and God's help that led to the giant's death.

Being intentional takes time, effort, and strategy. With God's help, you too can be intentional as you seek to glorify Him with your body. He's ready to give you victory, defeating your fitness foes and taking down the giants in your life.

Prayer

Father, thank You for David's example of a heart that chased yours. Will You please forgive me when mine doesn't? Please help me to be wise. May my words and actions be measured. Please help me consider the consequences of my actions beforehand. Amen.

Meditation

May I, by your help, be intentional in all areas of my life.

Daily Spiritual Exercise

God's provision, faithfulness, and power had each been manifested in David's life previously. As such, David was able to rely on these attributes of God during his confrontation with Goliath. Meditate on one of these attributes reflecting the "Bigness" of God today. As God did for David, God is more than able to provide your every need.

Week 2 Day 2 | *Old Testament Heroes: Job*

Of all the men and women in the Old Testament, Job may be the most underrated. He starts well, lives well, and ends well, with only a hiccup in between.

When we are first introduced to Job, no time is wasted in describing his character. Job 1:1 says, "This man was blameless and upright; he feared God and shunned evil." Then, two verses later, we learn, "He was the greatest man among all the people of the East." Wow! I'm not even the greatest man on the east side of my cul-de-sac.

God knew the strength of Job's character would sustain him when Satan was looking for someone to tear down. God allowed Satan to kill Job's children and destroy his immense wealth.

Job's response? Verses 20–22 say, "Then he fell to the ground in worship and said: 'Naked I came from my mother's womb, and naked I will depart. The Lord gave and the Lord has taken away; may the name of the Lord be praised.' In all this, Job did not sin by charging God with wrongdoing."

Satan then claimed Job's response was because his own life was spared. So again, God allowed Satan to harm Job, but not kill him. Satan afflicted Job with "painful sores from the soles of his feet to the crown of his head."

Even then, Job remains upright. His wife? Not so much: "His wife said to him, 'Are you still maintaining your integrity? Curse God and die!' He replied, 'You are talking like a foolish woman. Shall we accept good from God, and not trouble?' In all this, Job did not sin in what he said" (Job 2:9–10).

As if all this wasn't enough, three of Job's friends came to comfort him in his suffering. They started on the right track, merely weeping with him and not talking. However, the silence got the best of them. Chapters 3–37 detail the back and forth between Job and his buddies. They are unsupportive, insensitive, without empathy, and they even mischaracterize God. This is also when we find Job slipping some. He laments his birth, questions God's silence, and petitions for his own innocence.

The Lord reappears in Chapter 38 and, for a few chapters, takes Job to task for Job's various accusations. In Chapter 42, Job confesses:

"I know that you can do all things; no purpose of yours can be thwarted."—verse 2 (NIV)

The Lord is pleased with Job's response, but not so much Job's friends because they spoke untruths about God. In His mercy, God allows them to repent by sacrificing burnt offerings and accepting Job's prayer over their lives.

After all of this, Job's fortunes and family are more than restored. God blesses the latter part of Job's life more than the former part.

The Book of Job is ripe with lessons and encouragement. The next time you go through a trial, consider the possibility that you were specifically chosen for the task. Perhaps God ordained the circumstances because He wanted no one else but you to fulfill His purposes.

Speaking of purposes, we aren't always going to know the reason, nor do we need to. Job learned this the hard way. We need to learn to trust in the abundance of God's infinite wisdom that He knows what He's doing.

As you go about your fitness journey, you are going to have friends like Job who say unsupportive things: "Live a little," "You're a health nut," or "Don't get too skinny." People often speak out of their own insecurities and ignorance. Your example is convicting them, but they don't know how to handle it. You just need to maintain your focus.

You also need to maintain your integrity in . . . all . . . things. When you look back, you see that Job's first response to complete disaster was worship. Utter tragedy in Job's life resulted in unreserved worship in Job's heart. He understood that the source of all he had was from God, and knew to accept the bad with the good. He was quick to admit when he was wrong and was also quick to forgive those who had wronged him.

Finally, Job said to God, "I know you can do all things." *All things.* Not some things. Not a few things. Not parts of things. All things.

We will face trials. When we do, Job's example of faithfulness can encourage us. It also can remind us that, as Job understood quite well, God is in control of all things. "All" includes sustaining you as you work on your health. All includes being the source of your character and strength. All includes fulfilling His plan and purpose for your life . . . a purpose that cannot be thwarted!

Prayer

Father, thank You for Job's example. Will You forgive me when my response to my life's circumstances is filled with doubt, selfishness, or envy? Please help my default response in all things to be worship. Thank You for choosing me to help fulfill your plan. Amen.

Meditation

As Job was upright, keep me upright.

Daily Spiritual Exercise

He alone is sufficient to sustain you during any trial you face. He alone can comfort you during the hardest of times. He alone can empower you to fight the temptation to complain, run, or revolt. Meditate on one of these attributes, all of which reflect the "bigness" of God.

Week 2 Day 3 | *Old Testament Heroes: Daniel*

Daniel is one of the most inspiring figures in the Old Testament, and for good reason. He responds perfectly to an imperfect situation.

We are catching up to Daniel in chapter 6. At this moment, Daniel's jealous contemporaries concoct a plan to get him killed. They tricked the king into signing a ridiculous decree that required anyone who prayed to anyone other than King Darius to be thrown into a lion's den.

Daniel 6:10 says, "Now when Daniel learned that the decree had been published, he went home to his upstairs room where the windows opened toward Jerusalem. Three times a day he got down on his knees and prayed, giving thanks to his God, just as he had done before."

Therefore, Daniel's first response, in spite of his obstacles, was to pray and "give thanks." Notice also that he did this often . . . three times a day. Furthermore, this was nothing new for Daniel. The words "just as he had before" are evidence that He was a man characterized by a thankful heart. Daniel was a man devoted to God and prayer.

Daniel 6:11 says, "Then these men went as a group and found Daniel praying and asking God for help."

So here Daniel was, facing the possibility of becoming cat food. His default reaction? Give thanks regularly and ask God for help. He didn't set out to figure it out on his own. He set out for God.

The men, however, proceeded to rat on Daniel. We're told that King Darius had great anguish over this. In the end, though, he felt he was left with no choice but to feed Daniel to the lions.

First thing the next morning the king rushed to check on Daniel. After calling down to him, King Darius heard the following response:

> *"My God sent his angel, and he shut the mouths of the lions. They have not hurt me, because I was found innocent in his sight. Nor have I ever done any wrong before you, Your Majesty."* –Daniel 6:22 (NIV)

Because Daniel was innocent before God and man, God shut the mouths of the lions.

Daniel 6:23 reads, "The king was overjoyed and gave orders to lift Daniel out of the den. And when Daniel was lifted from the den, no wound was found on him, because he had trusted in his God."

Verse 26 continues, "I issue a decree that in every part of my kingdom people must fear and reverence the God of Daniel." The chapter concludes by telling us that Daniel prospered during the king's reign.

So let's look again at Daniel's reaction: he prayed regularly, gave thanks, asked for help, and trusted God.

God's response? He not only spared Daniel, but also elevated him while bringing glory back to himself.

My pastor tells a great story about visiting a woman from our church. As they were talking, he noticed a painting of Daniel in the lion's den. The woman asked my pastor if there was anything he liked about the depiction. After he mentioned a few things, the woman chimed in, "You know what I like? I like that Daniel isn't looking at the lions or his surroundings, nor does he seem worried. Instead, he's looking back up through the hole through which he was thrown. He's looking toward the sky, like he had so many times before as he prayed."

In the coming weeks of this fitness journey, it will be easy to look around at the lions we're facing. Healthy food we don't like. Junk food we do like. Making time to get adequate sleep. Finding time to plan ahead with our meal prep. Mustering the motivation to work out. Off-handed remarks from those around us. Insecurities about past failures.

Yet like Daniel in the painting and Daniel in real life, our focus should be only on our Father. Our response should be just like Daniel's:

We should pray regularly. Daily, three times a day, hourly, moment by moment.

We should give thanks. We may not like all we are working through, but we should give thanks in spite of it.

We should ask for help. Help with the desire, with the fortitude, with wisdom, and for the strength.

We should trust God. God is bigger than all this, more than able to help, and more than willing. We just need to be pure in our motives.

Make no mistake: lions are lying in wait. The temptation will be to worry about what they *might* do rather than on what the Lord *can* do.

If God can shut the mouths of hungry lions, He can certainly open the way for hearts hungry for Him.

Prayer
Father, thank You that You are a God who can be trusted to deliver me. Will You forgive me when I fear the lions rather than focus on You? Please help me keep my eyes on You at all times, trusting You with the outcome. Amen.

Meditation
God is bigger than lions.

Daily Spiritual Exercise
Daniel modeled prayer, thankfulness, and trust during a trial that could have scared him out of it. We would be wise to do the same with our fitness. So meditate on an attribute of God exemplifying how He delivers us during frightening times.

Week 2 Day 4 | *Old Testament Heroes: Abraham*

Abraham is known for many things. None may be more notable than his ultimate example of obedience when the Lord tested him:

> *"Then God said, 'Take your son, your only son, whom you love—Isaac—and go to the region of Moriah. Sacrifice him there as a burnt offering on a mountain I will show you.' Early the next morning Abraham got up and loaded his donkey. He took with him two of his servants and his son Isaac."—Genesis 22:2–3 (NIV)*

Okay, stop there. I'm not sure about you, but I'd certainly have questions. However, what do we see from Abraham? Obedience without question. God gives Abraham some horrifying instructions, and the next morning, early morning no less, Abraham responds with obedience. The story goes on:

> *"On the third day Abraham looked up and saw the place in the distance. He said to his servants, 'Stay here with the donkey while I and the boy go over there. We will worship and then we will come back to you.'"—Genesis 22:4–5 (NIV)*

Notice Abraham's complete obedience. He didn't choose a destination of his own. Instead, he went to "the place" on the mountain in Moriah, per the Lord's directions.

Also notice that Abraham says "we" will come back to you after worshipping, meaning he *and* Isaac. Abraham believed the Lord would salvage the situation. We see this faith displayed again when Isaac asks his dad where the lamb was:

> *"Abraham answered, 'God himself will provide the lamb for the burnt offering, my son.'"—Genesis 22:8 (NIV)*

After the altar was built, God still had not provided a lamb. At this point, if I'm Abraham, I'm facing a crisis of belief. *Where's the help? Where's the provision? Where's the relief?* Not Abraham. He continues in obedience:

"He bound his son Isaac and laid him on the altar, on top of the wood. Then he reached out his hand and took the knife to slay his son."—Genesis 22:9–10 (NIV)

Imagine the anguish and horror in that moment. Envision reconciling the internal conflict of sacrificing someone you love for someone you love more. Your knife is raised high and ready to cut short the life of someone so important to you.

Of course, we know the story doesn't end there. God interrupts:

"'Do not do anything to him. Now I know that you fear God, because you have not withheld from me your son, your only son.' Abraham looked up and there in a thicket he saw a ram caught by its horns. He went over and took the ram and sacrificed it as a burnt offering instead of his son. So Abraham called that place The Lord Will Provide."—Genesis 22:12–14 (NIV)

God came through, just as Abraham had expected. Not only did God provide, He then rewarded Abraham's obedience. Abraham would have "descendants as numerous as the stars in the sky and as the sand on the seashore."

I'm not sure what has led you to go on this fitness journey. Maybe you're sick and tired of being sick and tired. Maybe you've been healthy your whole life, but for the wrong reasons. Or maybe you feel prompted by the Lord to "sacrifice" your old ways. They're keeping you from complete obedience in all areas of your life. Whatever the case, it's important to establish a couple things early on.

First, while I know this journey can be scary, you need to expect that the Lord will provide. Yes, the mountain ahead is daunting and the work intimidates you. *What if it's too hard? What if you go back to your old ways? What if you can never establish a healthy body image?* Do not question the calling. Just trust and expect that the Lord will provide.

You also need to be ready to raise the knife if He doesn't make your fitness easier. He may never alleviate the burden of exercise. He may not provide a way out of the difficulty of eating healthy. There may be no ram in the thicket. You need to be ready to sacrifice some things you love for someone you love more. In spite of the results this yields, you need to be ready and willing.

Ultimately, the fitness results you may or may not see on Earth will be seen in heaven. Why? Because obedience is never wasted, and in God's kingdom, it never goes unrewarded.

Prayer
Father, thank You for all the ways You have provided for me already. Will You forgive me when I question your plans for me? Please help me be obedient to You in all things. Amen.

Meditation
I will trust and obey.

Daily Spiritual Exercise
The physical outcome we are hoping for with our fitness should not dictate our obedience. Abraham did not know the outcome, but he stayed obedient, trusting in God's provision. Meditate on His provision in your life today. This includes the provision to help you stay the course regardless of the results.

Week 2 Day 5 | *Old Testament Heroes: Solomon*

Imagine God comes to you at the beginning of your fitness journey. He says to you, "Ask for whatever you want me to give you."

How do you think you'd respond? "Help me to lose 43 pounds." "Help me to set a new PR in my upcoming marathon." "I would like a six-pack." "Can I please fit in my old clothes without exercising?" Those things are fine and dandy. However, I think the Lord would be more pleased by a different kind of answer . . . the kind that Solomon gave.

We pick up the story with a newly minted King Solomon. In 1 Kings 3:3 we read that Solomon had been showing "his love for the Lord by walking according to the instructions given him by his father David." Then, the Lord appears to Solomon. It happens one night after Solomon offers "a thousand burnt offerings" (verse 4) at the most important high place in Gibeon. Right off the bat, we find Solomon following his earthly father's instructions, walking with his heavenly Father, consistently obedient.

In the dream, God offers Solomon anything he wants. Verse 6 reads, "You have shown great kindness to your servant, my father David, because he was faithful to you and righteous and upright in heart." Before he asks for anything, he professes God's kindness and faithfulness.

Verse 7 continues, "But I am only a little child and do not know how to carry out my duties." Solomon shows his humility, acknowledging that he's in over his head. Verse 8 follows with, "Your servant is here among the people you have chosen, a great people, too numerous to count or number." Solomon continues his humility, but also acknowledges his role in God's plan: he is a servant. He exists to carry out God's plan.

Finally, Solomon makes his request. Verse 9 says, "So give your servant a discerning heart to govern your people and to distinguish between right and wrong." He reaffirms his servant role and asks for a discerning heart. Not riches. Not armies. Not land or power or anything else . . . only a discerning heart.

This pleased God a great deal, as we read in His response:

"I will give you a wise and discerning heart, so that there will never have been anyone like you, nor will there ever be. Moreover, I will give you what you have not asked for—both wealth and honor—so that in your lifetime you will have no equal among kings."—1 Kings 3:12–13 (NIV)

Let's recap. Solomon was obedient in his walk. He was grateful for God's faithfulness and kindness. He remained God's humble servant. In spite of his position as king and with some degree of wisdom already, Solomon asked for more. *He asks for what he needs, not what he wants.* He asked for a discerning heart.

Like Solomon, we want to be found obedient, grateful, humble, and willing to grow. Far too often, we work on our fitness for the things we want, not the things we need. However, if we stop, back up, and start over, we can reorient our approach. Therefore, don't pray, "God, please make that scale move today." Instead, pray, "God, help me find my comfort in you and not food today." Don't pray: "God, will you let me get my fastest time today at the race." Rather we can pray, "God, help me be smart as I'm running and more importantly, enjoy You while I do." Let's not approach Him with "Lord, I'd really like a six-pack." Instead, submit to Him. "Lord, I can do no good thing apart from You . . . help me to keep You the main thing." Let's not complain with "Lord, I don't want to exercise." He already knows this. Instead, pray, "Father, You know that I struggle with being active, but I know You can change that. I'm open to wherever you lead me because I know I need to move more."

Notice that Solomon didn't pray that the Lord would give him obedient people . . . he didn't pray for a result. Solomon prayed for discernment. He prayed for the ability to distinguish between right and wrong. He didn't pray for the destination. He prayed to be equipped for the journey.

When we have a discerning heart, we too are better equipped. When we know what to pray for, we can pray in such a way that it brings God glory. In a way, that will help us bring Him honor as we work on our health. In a way, that helps us focus on behaviors and not results.

Be discerning in how you approach the God of all creation with your requests. Ultimately, God doesn't care about your six-pack, but He does care about your heart . . . so pray for a discerning one.

Prayer

Father, thank You that I can come to You with anything. Will You forgive me when I'm concerned about the wrong things? Please give this servant of Yours a discerning heart and the ability to distinguish wants from needs. Amen.

Meditation

You are the source of my wisdom.

Daily Spiritual Exercise

Wisdom is not overrated. We would be wise to pursue it with all our hearts, as it will guide our fitness and beyond. God is the provider of that wisdom as He is wisdom Himself. Meditate on that attribute of His character today.

Week 2 Day 6 | *Old Testament Heroes: The "Here I Ams"*

At not quite three, my son Silas is old enough to play games around the house. However, he's not old enough to fully understand the premise. Playing tag, for instance, can result in him running toward me rather than away. Soccer frequently involves more hands than feet. Just try playing the generational favorite, hide-and-seek. One of the children counts to ten. A tucked-away Silas hears the "Ready or not, here I come." Instantly, a distant "Here I am" can be heard coming from Mommy and Daddy's closet. Good try, buddy, but you're it . . . again.

Silas would have fit right in with many of our favorite men from the Old Testament. "Here I am" was a frequent response from many of the greats. In fact, it was the perfect response, though it seems a little unusual on the surface.

For instance, the testing of Abraham in Genesis begins with God saying Abraham's name and Abraham replying, "Here I am." Later on in the same chapter, before the knife drops, we read:

> *"But the angel of the Lord called out to him from heaven, 'Abraham! Abraham!' 'Here I am,' he replied."—Genesis 22:11 (NIV)*

Two different times, in Genesis 31 and in Genesis 46, God calls to Jacob in a dream. Both times, Jacob answers, "Here I am."

When God called out to Moses from within the famous burning bush, Moses said, "Here I am."

Samuel used this phrase four times. The first three times God called, Samuel mistakenly responded to Eli instead, with, "Here I am." Finally, the morning after God had shared the vision with Samuel, he got it right. Eli called for him. Samuel came to him, saying yet again "Here I am." The fourth time is a charm.

There's a lot we can learn from these men and their default answers. Now, at first glance, "Here I am" might seem like a strange thing to say. This wasn't Silas playing hide-and-seek. It wasn't as if God didn't know where they were. "Here I am" was really a way of acknowledging their availability, not their geographical location. "Here I am" could be read, "I'm here, fully available for you."

Secondly, in order for them to respond, they needed to be listening in the first place. Like Silas in the closet, ears open, eager to engage, these men were open to hearing from God. Not at a specific time, but at all times. Due to Eli's prompting, when God called for Samuel for the fourth time, Samuel responded, "Your servant is listening."

Lastly, whenever we see God's people obediently behaving in similar ways, we can take that as a cue. We can learn from them and apply it in our own lives.

What if we applied the "Here I am" mindset to our fitness? Maybe you are already doing that . . . you're reading this book, after all. Even still, you may be reading this reluctantly. Another area of your life might be easier to turn over to God—your money, job, free time—but fitness, not so much. You're semi-available.

Perhaps you're available to Him physically because you know you should be exercising and eating healthy, so you do. Yet in your heart of hearts, you haven't truly turned it over to Him. You're just going through the motions. You're available, just not quite fully.

Maybe you have this nudging deep in your spirit that you're trying to tune out. However, that could very well be the Holy Spirit churning in you. He's trying to cultivate a complete surrender of every part of you. If you're pulling a Moses, trying to avoid it at all costs, it's time to relent. It's time to reply, "Here I am."

Maybe you've refused to open your ears to listen to *all* He might be revealing to you. Perhaps you're not listening . . . through Scripture, your prayer life, through quiet times, your friendship base, or your circumstances. If you are not listening, you could be missing out on the Lord's blessings.

Remember, every time the Lord spoke to His people and they responded with "Here I am," one of three things happened: they were blessed, they were used by God, and/or they were blessed by being used by God.

What if being attentive and available in every area of our lives could result in being used by God? "Here I am" is suddenly not such a strange response at all. In fact, it's the perfect response. Because you know what?

Ready or not, here He comes.

Prayer

Father, thank You for wanting to use me. Will You forgive me when I'm not listening or refuse to make myself available? Please work on my heart in this way so that I might bring You glory. Amen.

Meditation

I'm listening and I'm available.

Daily Spiritual Exercise

God honors availability, including our availability with our fitness. So meditate on an attribute of God that will help you remain available—maybe His consistency, steadfastness, provision, or comfort. Whichever attribute helps you stay open to His leading, meditate on it and pray it over your life.

Week 2 Day 7 | *Old Testament Heroes: Manoah and His Wife*

"Ma-who-a?"

If you had to look it up in your Bible or Google it, I wouldn't blame you. Manoah was Samson's father.

While Samson was famous for his strength, you'll find that his parents were far more impressive than he was. In fact, Samson lived a more "here's what not to do" kind of life. Taking a closer look at his parents reveals an attitude and approach we can apply to our lives.

Judges 13 starts with a familiar refrain, "Again the Israelites did evil in the eyes of the Lord." However, in God's great grace, He had a plan to restore His people. Through Manoah and his wife (we never learn her name), God would bring up Samson, an Israelite judge for 20 years.

We read next that an angel of the Lord appears to Manoah's barren wife. The angel, whose divine identity was lost on her at first, tells her she would have a son. The angel had very specific instructions for them. They were not to have wine or fermented drink, eat anything unclean, or ever cut Samson's hair.

When Manoah's wife tells her husband what happened, he responds:

> *"Pardon your servant, Lord. I beg you to let the man of God you sent to us come again to teach us how to bring up the boy who is to be born." –Judges 13:8 (NIV)*

Manoah doesn't question why these things are happening. He doesn't try to pass the buck to someone else (Exodus 4:13). Manoah simply seeks God's help for God's instructions. He's never told that Samson would be given incredible strength. He just knows that a responsibility has been placed in his path. Therefore, he immediately seeks God's help in carrying out God's will.

We too would be wise to first seek God. We need His help in determining how to carry out His will for our health. Too often, even though we know we're supposed to do something, we don't include God in the process. If we've determined it's God's will to honor Him with our bodies, shouldn't we ask Him how we should do this? Wouldn't it make more sense to seek His help for something we've concluded He has commanded? Manoah certainly would think so.

God listens to Manoah's request. Manoah asks the angel, "When your words are fulfilled, what is to be the rule that governs the boy's life and work?" (verse 8).

Notice there is no doubt in Manoah's voice: "When your words are fulfilled." He doesn't question the authenticity, validity, or potential for success of the angel's prediction. He trusts that what is said will happen.

When the Lord gives us instructions, how do we respond? Do we lace our obedience in reluctance and doubt? Or does the strength of conviction lead us to take action? Do we dip our toes in the fitness waters, while deep down inside wondering what good it will do? Do we dive in headfirst, focusing on behaviors and trusting God to take care of the results? Again, we know what Samson's parents would do.

After the angel answers them, they respond with a heart of gratitude by offering the angel dinner. While it would be a great honor to be the parents of an Israelite leader, it's not like they're suddenly living on easy street. In fact, their personal responsibility in the matter has increased; the stakes have been raised. Yet out of a heart of thanksgiving, they want to give back.

It would be prudent for us to live our lives in a permanent state of gratefulness as well. The Lord has done so much for us. While our personal responsibilities may have to grow, we also can respond with a heart of appreciation. It's a marvel that the Lord would even want to be involved in our lives on every level.

The angel refused dinner, but suggested that they present a burnt offering to the Lord instead. Manoah and his wife took a goat and grain offering and sacrificed it to the Lord. That was when the angel's true identity was revealed.

When we're asked to give what we perceive is a sacrifice, our real identity, our true nature is revealed too. For some of us, our fitness is too big to turn over to God. For others, it's so small that we deem it not important enough to present to God. God, however, wants to be not just involved, but in charge of all areas of our lives, big and small.

So, do we believe that God wants to be involved in all areas of our lives, including our fitness? If so, Manoah and his wife give us a wonderful blueprint to follow: seek God's help, trust Him with the outcome, and follow through with a heart of appreciation.

We may never know how God might use our "fitness offerings" for His will. We do know that all our offerings can reveal the priorities of our hearts.

Although Samson's power was impressive, it pales in comparison to the spiritual strength of a heart powered by God.

Prayer
Father, thank You for Manoah and his wife's example. Will You forgive me when I react with my efforts, my distrust, and my reluctance? Please help me rely on You to determine and supply my needs.

Meditation
What You require, You provide.

Daily Spiritual Exercise
Seeking help, trusting God, and having gratitude with your fitness will go a long way toward empowering it. Meditate on an attribute of God (His grace, power, sufficiency) that best helps insure that you're doing these things.

WEEK 3 PREVIEW
Names for God

Our human nature tends to default to relying on ourselves for the source of most everything. This can be especially true of acts requiring our bodies. I'm not just talking exercise. We get hungry and so we eat. We wake up tired, so we drink coffee, tea, or soda. We're tired at the end of the day. However, we plow through a little while longer with little regard to the fact that our bodies need to sleep. We don't often pause to consider who God is during times like this. We don't always rely on the Holy Spirit to help us live healthier lives.

The better we understand the character of God, the better He can help us with our fitness. With that in mind, this week we're focusing on seven of the many, many ways God reveals His character throughout Scripture. Each of these names of God serves as a reminder of who He is and what He has done. They should also encourage us regarding what *He can do for us and through us* over the remaining 74 days. We need to allow Him to change our default. No more relying on us—we need to rely on Him as the source of everything . . . including our fitness.

Daily Spiritual Exercise: Sing a song of praise.
Isaiah 42:10 says, "Sing to the Lord a new song, his praise from the ends of the earth, you who go down to the sea, and all that is in it, you islands, and all who live in them."

Every day this week, by yourself, listen to a praise song and belt out worship to our great God. If you don't know the lyrics, print them off or find them online. I prefer to have headphones on and crank up the volume to drown out my own voice. I'm completely serious. You need to be by yourself. You need to sing out loud, whatever song gets your heart thumping, hands clapping, feet tapping, and spirit racing.

You are singing for an audience of one and you are glorifying Him in the heavens.

Week 3 Day 1 | *Names for God: The Potter*

The Bible uses several descriptions to depict God as the creative and masterful designer He is. Peter refers to him as "Creator" (1 Peter 4:19). In Job and the Psalms, God is mentioned as "Maker" (Job 35:10; Psalm 95:6). Of course, God's own son, Jesus, was by trade a carpenter, the very essence of a craftsman.

In my mind, no term better captures the image of a creator than that of a potter:

> *"Yet you, Lord, are our Father. We are the clay, you are the potter; we are all the work of your hand."—Isaiah 64:8 (NIV)*

Think about the creative process of potters. They start with clay. If you've ever held clay, you know there's nothing remarkable about it. It's a lump. Lifeless. Cold and dull.

Then the potters do something quite extraordinary. With only their hands and imagination, water and a wheel, they turn the clay into the vessel of their choosing: a fluted vase, a serving bowl, a water pitcher, a cup, or a statue.

A few things strike me about this imagery.

First, the clay does nothing on its own. It doesn't wake up one day and decide it will be a bowl, and poof . . . it's a bowl! It may want to be a bowl, but it will remain a mound of clay until the potter is finished.

We, too, can do no good things on our own. David says in Psalm 16:2, "I say to the Lord, 'You are my Lord; apart from you I have no good thing.'" Apart from our Creator, our Potter, we can do no good thing.

Secondly, no two pieces of pottery are perfectly identical. There may be lots of cups that are the same size, same shape, even painted the same color. Still, they're not exactly the same.

Neither are we, nor should we long to be. Imagine a plate saying to the potter, "I want to be a vase. Pour some water in me and I'll hold beautiful flowers." The water would run everywhere and the flowers would flop, withering even faster. The plate would fail because that wasn't the potter's design for it. We are all different, made unique for a reason, a specific purpose.

Early in a fitness journey, there is optimism, hope, visions of change and opportunity, as well there should be. It's exciting! We will need to remember, draw on, and channel that fervor throughout the coming weeks. It won't always be there . . . emotions come and go.

However, God—our Creator, our Potter—is steadfast. He is unchanging. His strength will always be there for us. We'll need Him, because apart from Him, we can do no good thing.

Furthermore, the journey and destination will be far more fulfilling when we understand that we're all made differently. God has an ordained purpose specific to us. If you're a plate, don't envy a vase. If you're a vase, don't boast; there's plenty the plate can do that you can't.

Lastly, you need to allow Him to work on you during this time; not just physically, but spiritually and emotionally. Listen for what He's trying to teach you. If He bends you this way or that way, go with it. If you resist, if you become stiff and stubborn, you'll dry out, crack and crumble in the process.

On the other hand, if you stay malleable, humble and open to His leading, He will create a masterpiece out of you. After all, we are the works of His hands. The Potter made you "you" for a reason and He does not make mistakes. He never stops or gives up on us. He continues to form us into an image that, day by day, looks more and more like His Son.

Never forget: God is the pre-eminent artist. As an artist, He has a vision for the shape of your future.

Trust the Potter's hands.

Prayer

Thank You for thinking so much of me, for creating me, for the purposes You have in mind for me. Will You forgive me when I'm unsatisfied with who You created me to be? Please guide, direct, and sustain me because without You, I can do no good thing. Amen."

Meditation

You are the potter; I'm the clay.

Daily Spiritual Exercise

Sing a song of praise.

Week 3 Day 2 | *Names for God: Breath of Life*

Most of us are familiar with John 14:6, where Jesus says, "I am the way and the truth and the life. No one comes to the Father except through me." In other words, no one can have eternal life with the Father, except through His son, Jesus.

However, have you ever stopped to consider that God is life itself? Not so much that He created life, though He did. Not that because of Him we have lives to live, though we do.

It's much more than that. God himself *is* life by His very nature. Then, out of that same nature, He gives us life.

Can you think of anyone who both gives life and is life? An animator brings motions to a static drawing, but is not life itself. A mechanic builds an engine that powers cars, boats, and planes, but is not life itself. A gardener tends to barren land from which plants grow, but is not life itself.

A more fitting analogy might be the elements. The ocean gives us water and is water itself. The sky gives us air and is air itself. The sun gives light and is light itself. The source of the attribute and the attribute itself are one and the same.

However, on their own, even the elements would be lifeless were it not for God. Without His touch, the ocean would be motionless, the sky an empty void, the sun merely a ball of gas.

This is all established in the beginning:

> *"Then the Lord God formed a man from the dust of the ground and breathed into his nostrils the breath of life, and the man became a living being."—Genesis 2:7 (NIV)*

The first part of the verse says, "Then the Lord God formed a man from the dust of the ground." At this point, God has created man. Also at this point, man has no life. He . . . just . . . is. Like a balloon without the helium, the man has no purpose or function.

Later in verse 7, God says "and breathed into his nostrils the breath of life, and the man became a living being." Man went from a thing to a being with merely a breath from God.

God is not just the giver of life. God is life.

Exercise is a privilege, not a sacrifice. If you're sore from yesterday's workout, it's probably hard to see it that way. After all, it's easy to take for granted the amazing intricacies of our bodies. At any given time, without a moment's thought, your body is doing thousands of things simultaneously. Cells are reproducing, axons and dendrites are working in sync, and the heart is pumping. Food is digesting, pupils are dilating and constricting, and the pituitary gland is regulating hormones. Kidneys are filtering blood, muscles contracting and expanding, ears processing sound waves, and on and on and on. None of this requires any thought from you.

It all originates from the Breath of Life. By His breath your cells are held together. By His breath your synapses are firing. By His breath your lungs are filling. By His breath your heart is beating.

As the steward of the body God has entrusted to you, look for ways to bring Him glory. Don't just praise Him *with* your body, but praise Him *for* it. Worship Him for the life He gave you and for the life He breathed into you.

Then take joy in the honor to be included in His plan.

Prayer
God, thank You. Your design is perfect. Will You forgive me for ever being a poor steward of the life You have given me? Please allow the Holy Spirit in me to bring glory to You with the body You have entrusted to me. Amen.

Meditation
You don't just give life. You are life.

Daily Spiritual Exercise
Sing a song of praise.

Week 3 Day 3 | *Names for God: Father*

If God created us, it would then make sense to consider Him our Father, would it not? Jesus often referred to God as His father. In fact, Jesus instructed us to pray to Him this way, in what's commonly known as "The Lord's Prayer":

> *"This, then, is how you should pray: 'Our Father in heaven, hallowed be your name.'"–Matthew 6:9 (NIV)*

In fact, we can learn a lot from the Lord's Prayer, not only what it means to have a father, but to have *our* Father.

Our Father is worthy of our respect, as shown in verse 9: "hallowed be your name." "Hallowed" isn't a word we use often, but it means to be considered holy and sacred. As a father of four, I certainly require respect from my children. How much more should we respect our Father, who, unlike us, is inherently holy?

A father's role also includes that of a "provider." Verse 11 says, "Give us today our daily bread." I feel the beautiful burden of being the provider for our family. I consider it a privilege to make sure their needs are met, that they are fed, clothed, and warm. That said, they also have emotional and spiritual needs that need to be addressed, cultivated, and nurtured. Our Father does the same for us, only He does it perfectly. As verse 12 indicates, only He can provide our forgiveness.

A father also is a leader, as we see in verse 17 when Jesus says, "Lead us not into temptation." It's far easier to avoid temptation than to prevail in the face of it. I want to put my children in a place to succeed. Part of the way to do this is by leading them clear of situations where temptation is lurking. We, too, would be wise to rely on the Father for direction and guidance in all areas of our lives.

When I think about my duties as a father, the first one that comes to mind is "protector." At night, I'm the one who makes sure the doors are locked. When putting a car seat in, I double-check that it's secured correctly. When the kids want to watch TV, my first thought is to make sure it's safe programming. If they were ever attacked in my presence, I would protect them. Our Father is our protector as well, as we see at the conclusion of the Lord's Prayer. Jesus says, "deliver us from the evil one." The fact is we can't avoid all temptation. Fortunately, our Protector-Father has a remedy for that as well . . . as we submit to Him in our trials, He can deliver us from them.

These attributes of a father serve us well as we seek to take care of our bodies. Again, God deserves our respect. That respect should manifest itself in our words and deeds. That includes respecting these bodies He created and into which he breathes life. Don't be fooled, though. Over-exercising is not showing respect, nor is under-sleeping because you're so busy "serving the kingdom." (Youth ministers especially need to be on guard against this.)

If you're living in the United States, our Father has already provided an incredible abundance of healthy foods. Yes, eating healthier can be more expensive, but so is living better in general. Furthermore, there are gyms everywhere, corporate wellness facilities, in-home workout programs, and of course the great outdoors. Exercise options are literally a step away.

At first, asking the Father to lead our fitness lives might seem like a strange request. However, our Father doesn't want us to struggle with this any more than I want my children to struggle when they're earnestly seeking answers. So, seek His leadership. James 1:5–6 tells us not only to pray for wisdom, but to expect an answer. If you're struggling for wisdom with your fitness, pray and expect God to deliver. Then, when He does, be honest enough to recognize Him and accept His leading. Those nudges that will undoubtedly come your way are not a coincidence.

Unfortunately, living healthy lives doesn't guarantee we will stay healthy. Injuries are routine and disease happens, which is one reason why we want to pray for protection. We also don't want to rely solely on our own physical efforts, thereby removing our need for the Lord's leadership. As Proverbs 3:6 instructs, we want to acknowledge Him in *all* our ways.

When we put our Father first, and rely on His provision and protection, we can rest assured that His will . . . will be done.

Prayer

God, thank You for the abundance in my life, which all comes from You. Will You forgive me when I try to lead myself rather than rely on You? Please give me wisdom and protection as I seek to glorify You with the body You have given to me. Amen.

Meditation

You are not just a father, but You are my perfect Father.

Daily Spiritual Exercise

Sing a song of praise.

Week 3 Day 4 | *Names for God: Dwelling Place*

When the term "dwelling place" is used in Scripture, usually it's referring to a residence. Makes sense. It would also make sense that when we consider God's dwelling place, we would naturally think about heaven. In fact, we see the term used that way in Solomon's prayer in 1 Kings 8, where he says, "Hear from heaven, your dwelling place." In verse 30, 39, 43 and 49, as well as many times in 2 Chronicles, Solomon refers to heaven.

David, in Psalm 33:13–14, says, "From heaven the Lord looks down and sees all mankind; from his dwelling place he watches, all who live on earth."

Later, the meaning changes . . . and I love it:

> *"Lord, you have been our dwelling place throughout all generations."*
> *—Psalm 90:1 (NIV)*

"Dwelling place" has shifted from describing a location to describing a person . . . the person of the Lord. This is significant for at least two reasons.

First of all, David is implying that the Lord Himself is home . . . our home. As we read in the very next verse, it has always been this way: "Before the mountains were born or you brought forth the whole world, from everlasting to everlasting you are God." So, even before the world was, the Lord has been our home.

Something else is noteworthy about the Lord being our dwelling place. When we profess Him as Lord and invite Him to live in our hearts, we become a dwelling place for Him. 1 Corinthians 6:19 states, "Do you not know that your bodies are temples of the Holy Spirit, who is in you, whom you have received from God? You are not your own." We are in Him and He is in us. Imagine! The one who hung the sun, moon, and stars would want to live in our hearts. We should be humbled.

If I were to be completely honest, I could not say that He is always my dwelling place. My sinful nature creeps in and my heart wants what it wants. My mind wanders. My strength or hope or peace is coming from the wrong source. It's coming from my miserable cup of humanity rather than His endless well of perfection.

Perhaps you've experienced this as well. More specifically, you've experienced it with your fitness. You see, when we are focused on the junk food we are giving up, we're not dwelling in Him. When we adopt a mindset of dread because exercising is hard, He is not our dwelling place. When we feel sorry for ourselves because we don't look like so and so, He is not our dwelling place. When we're absorbed with the struggle, rather than with the promises of His word, He is not our dwelling place.

The good news is it doesn't have to be this way. We need to be willing to allow Him to change us on the inside . . . to transform us emotionally and spiritually.

Remember that God living in us means we *should want* to dwell in Him. The more we are there, the less we want to be anywhere else.

Furthermore, He is perfection and I can do no good thing apart from Him. I don't just desire Him to be . . . *I need* Him to be my dwelling place.

Finally, it should not be surprising that He would want our hearts to be more like His. After all, He's living in them. He helps us, as when we notice our demeanor starting to shift inward instead of upward. That gentle nudge is a reminder to rely on Him as our dwelling place. That is God at work!

When we are living in and by Him, when our home is in His heart and He is in ours, things change. Our failures are no longer our focus. Our Father is.

There's no better dwelling place.

Prayer

Lord, thank You for wanting to reside in a sinner like me. Will You forgive me when I look outside of You for my source of strength or worth? Please give me a heart that only feels at home in You. Amen.

Meditation

You are my Dwelling Place.

Daily Spiritual Exercise

Sing a song of praise.

Week 3 Day 5 | *Names for God: Redeemer*

Every year, a couple of songs seem to resonate with me in a special way. It takes the right combination of a melody echoing the theme of the lyrics. When this happens, it grabs me by the shoulders and shakes me. "Beautiful Things" by Gungor has done just that.

If you're unfamiliar with that song, I'd encourage you to track it down. Then, close your eyes and give it a listen. Somehow, it's both melancholy and upbeat. It's honest as it speaks to the struggles, pain, and questions we face. It's also powerful as it reminds us of what Christ can do with us, in spite of our failings.

The first verse of "Beautiful Things" says:

> *All this pain*
> *I wonder if I'll ever find my way*
> *I wonder if my life could really change at all*

Have you ever felt this way about your fitness? You've tried and tried and tried and still can't seem to get a handle on it. You start strong, but fade just as fast. Food is a constant battle. Energy is never there for long. Your attitude, outlook, or worth is based on the scale. In fact, this book might be your last try at the whole fitness thing. You have simply come to the point where you wonder if you will ever find your way . . . if you will ever change.

Or maybe your doubt extends beyond fitness. Perhaps you are concerned if He can make much out of your life. It has certainly crossed my mind. For me, it's never so much an indictment on His ability to do so, but in His interest in doing so. "Me, Lord? Why would you want me when I've failed You so many times? There are far better people who could have a far greater impact than me. Besides, I haven't changed much up to this point . . . not sure if it will ever happen."

Then, the chorus to "Beautiful Things" reminds us:

> *You make beautiful things*
> *You make beautiful things out of the dust*
> *You make beautiful things*
> *You make beautiful things out of us*

Our Lord specializes not only in making beautiful things, but does so where no hint of beauty can be found.

In Genesis, we read that He breathed life into dust and there was man. Later, we read that, in spite of Joseph's brothers' wicked hearts, the Lord elevated Joseph to great prominence.

In Acts, we read how the Lord transformed Saul of Tarsus. Saul had previously brought great persecution to the Christian church. The Lord then turned him into one of the most influential Christians the world has known. Of course, in the ultimate restoration story, the Lord gave us Jesus. He sent His only Son to earth to pay the price of the cumulative sin of mankind.

So who can do such things? Who can change it all? Who can turn dark to light? Death to life? Only a Redeemer can. Only our Redeemer can:

> *"The Lord, your Redeemer who made you, says: 'All things were made by me; I alone stretched out the heavens. By myself I made the earth and everything in it.'"*—Isaiah 44:24 (TLB)

The Lord is not Lord in part. He is Lord of all. He has made everything that is without any help from anyone . . . anywhere . . . anytime . . . ever. That is who we have as our Redeemer! If He can do that, He certainly can make beautiful things out of us, our fitness included.

What's also exciting is that He has no interest in where we've been in the past, after we acknowledge our sin. We've acknowledged our need for His Son to save us. We've acknowledged that we can do no good thing apart from Him. Out of that recognition and confession of our weakness, God makes beautiful things.

You are nearly three weeks into this fitness journey. Doubts can start to arise—doubts based on your past. Will this time be any different? Can it last? Can you find your way? Can you truly change?

Unlike us, though, God doesn't see our past failings as obstacles or as indicators of future results. He sees what's possible because of the Holy Spirit at work within us.

Our fitness, like our faith, is a process. That process requires remembering and relying on the fact that God is working on us and in us. No matter our fitness past, He is making us beautiful and we should be overjoyed.

So, throughout the nine-ish weeks remaining, remember that with our Redeemer, hope is alive! As "Beautiful Things" concludes:

You make me new, You are making me new. You make me new, You are making me new.

Prayer
Father, thank You that because of the redemptive nature of who You are, we always have hope. Will You forgive me when I question what You can or will do with me? Please help me to trust your plan for my life. Thank You for making me . . . new.

Meditation
You are my Redeemer.

Daily Spiritual Exercise
Sing a song of praise.

Week 3 Day 6 | *Names for God: Lord of Hosts*

In your greatest moment of need, to whom do you turn?

If it's a basketball game and the score is tied, you give the ball to your best player. If there's medical trauma from a car crash, you turn to the ER doctors. Or if you're in war facing enemy fire, you rely on your commanding officer. You try to put your trust in those with the most ability, the most knowledge, or the most authority.

If we believe those we trust have any of these traits, the more we believe we improve our chances of victory. Unfortunately, nobody on earth perfectly exemplifies even one of these characteristics, let alone all of them. That's a job suited for the "Lord of Hosts."

Of the many names God gives Himself, there is none more prevalent than "Lord of Hosts." Depending on which Bible translation you read, you can see the term nearly 300 times. It first appears in 1 Samuel 1:3 with Elkanah, whose claim to fame was being Samuel's father.

Elkanah makes his annual trip to Shiloh to sacrifice to the "Lord of Hosts." We see it again in Isaiah 9, in the closing sentence of the most well known of the messianic prophecies, "For to Us a Child Is Born." Perhaps most famously, we see this phrase in David's rebuking of Goliath before David disposes of the giant:

> *"Then David said to the Philistine, 'You come to me with a sword and with a spear and with a javelin, but I come to you in the name of the Lord of hosts, the God of the armies of Israel, whom you have defied.'"—1 Samuel 17:45 (ESV)*

For all its frequency, this name for God is possibly the most nebulous of His descriptions. We may sing it in a hymn or read it in the Book of Psalms; however, we probably give little thought to what it really means, much less what it means for our quest for fitness.

When the name "Lord of Hosts" is used in the Bible (translated from the Hebrew "Jehovah Sabaoth"), "hosts" is generally meant in the military sense. It can be interpreted as "armies," probably to armies of angels. Some would also argue that the term refers to stars and other heavenly bodies. Both are true in the sense that God, the ultimate and final authority, commands them all. Everything in heaven and on earth is under the universal sovereignty of the Lord of Hosts.

When we're facing a crisis, our first response should be to turn to the Lord of Hosts. Yes, God has put people in our lives to minister to us and speak truth into our hearts. There are wonderful books that can unveil facets of the Christian life that previously were a mystery to us. Certainly, there are songs that raise spirits; sermons that can teach lessons; and websites that share testimonies of God's grace. These are all good things, but they're not the best as a first response.

The correct first response is to turn to God. Remember, He doesn't just have "the most" ability, knowledge, and authority. He has *all* the ability, knowledge, and authority to accomplish what He wills. So, by turning first to Him, we increase the likelihood of victory in the situation.

Furthermore, by looking to the Lord of Hosts first, we *guarantee* we will bring Him glory and honor. That alone is a victory.

This fitness journey will present many opportunities to seek things other than the Lord of Hosts in our moments of need: food, TV, people, sleep, books, websites, movies, drinks, activity, leisure, and so on. None of these things, however, will endure, satisfy, or fulfill.

In every moment of need, we can rely on the Lord of Hosts to keep his covenant with us. We can cry out, run to, sing for, call on, pray to, reach for, and side with our Warrior-God. Only He reverses inevitable defeat, returns lost hope, and redeems lost people.

Don't underestimate the power of having the Lord of Hosts empower you or you will settle for far too little. He has the knowledge to fulfill the prophecy of the birth of King Jesus. He has the authority to command armies of angels. He has the ability to deliver David from Goliath. The Lord of Hosts can deliver you too.

Prayer

Father, thank You that no single name can completely capture the fullness of Your character. Will You forgive me when I call on anyone other than You for my deliverance? Please help me to look to Your authority, ability, and knowledge as my first response. Amen.

Meditation

My Lord is also the Lord of Hosts.

Daily Spiritual Exercise

Sing a song of praise.

Week 3 Day 7 | *Names for God: God of Rest*

When I tell people that fitness is composed of three things, they generally know the first two: exercise and nutrition. However, when I tell them that the third factor determining their overall level of fitness is sleep, they seemed surprised. Sleep is for lazy people, right? Who has time to rest anyway? It's so unproductive . . . or is it?

The benefits of sleep fall into two categories, the first being the physiological functions. Your body does countless, incredible things when you're asleep. For instance, hormones are being regulated. Big deal, you say? Hormones are essential for muscle growth and development. Hormones help determine appetite satiation. Hormones are used to manage stress and control energy production sources and increase alertness.

Your tissue growth and repair occur in your sleep. Energy is restored. Your immune system is bolstered. Muscles relax, repair, and grow. The cardiovascular system gets a break with a lower heart rate and a drop in blood pressure. Toxic metabolic byproducts are removed from the brain. Memories are preserved. The list goes on and on, all happening without you even having to try.

Equally important are the emotional benefits of sleep. When well rested, you increase your ability to focus, lower your stress, and have a more positive demeanor. Getting good sleep will improve your decision-making process, including options regarding food and exercise. It's a whole lot easier to make bad nutrition choices when you have no energy. When we're low on energy, if we exercise at all, it often results in half-hearted efforts and a decreased benefit. Being tired usually results in poor decisions, rationalization, quick fixes, or unrealistic assumptions about how we'll do the next day.

When it's spelled out like this, it's easy to see why sleep is so important for your fitness. In a nutshell, it helps you repair and prepare, without you even having to try.

The Bible says that God formed us (Psalm 119:73). He made the delicate, inner parts of our body and knitted us together in our mother's womb

(Psalm 139:13). So, it should come as no surprise that the God of our bodies is also the God of rest. He did invent rest, after all:

> *"On the seventh day God had finished his work of creation, so he rested from all his work. And God blessed the seventh day and declared it holy, because it was the day when he rested from all his work of creation."—Genesis 2:2–3 (NLT)*

Now in fairness, rest and sleep are not always synonymous. God, of course, never sleeps (Psalm 121:4), but He has wired our bodies to require it. Furthermore, He has blessed us with permission to relax, recoup, and refresh for our days ahead. He has made it appropriate for us to repair and prepare.

God is also the God of a different kind of rest, as His Son tells us in Matthew:

> *"Then Jesus said, "Come to me, all of you who are weary and carry heavy burdens, and I will give you rest."—Matthew 11:28 (NLT)*

This kind of rest frees us from the compulsion to use our own strength to fix something we can't fix. We no longer need to keep trying, doing, and working for something that's already been offered through grace by faith. This kind of rest relinquishes us from the feeling that we must earn our deliverance. This kind of rest restores our souls for all of eternity. This is salvation rest.

The good news doesn't end there. The same assurance of being united with God in the someday allows us to go to Him in the now. The exhaustion we have in our earthly life, the loads we are carrying, the busyness, the problems and hardships—we can lay all this at His feet. The confidence and security that are born out of a relationship with Him serves only to lighten our load. He can replace Martha's work with Mary's wonder (Luke 10:38–42). God lets us rest in green meadows (Psalm 23:2). He invites us to experience rest that He prepared for us and promised to us (Hebrews 4:1–3).

Having 20 days of the fitness journey under your belt, you're hopefully realizing the benefits of your nightly sleep. It plays out in your workouts, the day's events, your decisions, and in your progress. Making it a priority will make the journey not only more rewarding, but more enjoyable.

The greatest need, however, is to fully rest in Him every step along the way. We need not worry or have anxiety about our fitness. We can relax. Exhale. Trust. For when we go to Him (as He teaches), we find rest for our souls (as He promises) because He does the work. Just as with our sleep at night, we are the ones who benefit and we don't even have to try.

Prayer
Thank You God for the gift of sleep and, even more so, for the gift of spiritual rest. Will You forgive me when I rest my efforts in anyone or anything other than You? Please help me to slow down, try less, and rest more. Amen.

Meditation
I will rest in Him.

Daily Spiritual Exercise
Sing a song of praise.

The King of "Un"

I f I described someone as strong, smart, and considerate, that probably sounds like someone you wouldn't mind calling a friend.

However, what if I described someone as unstoppable, unparalleled, and unflinching? Is there much you wouldn't do to have them in your corner?

Of all the words used to describe God, those beginning with "un" seem closest to doing Him justice:

- Unchanging
- Uncompromising
- Unending
- Unbiased
- Unfailing
- Unconventional
- Unassailable
- Unrelenting

Indeed, He is the King of "Un."

When you stop to think about serving a leader like God, do you feel empowered? Not because of anything you do, but because of who He is. With that power comes comfort. Assurance. Confidence.

Week 4 in a fitness program can present some obstacles. The newness and excitement that come with a fresh beginning have worn off. You start understanding that fitness as a short-term project will get you short-term results. That's discouraging. It's daunting to realize that a healthy lifestyle takes long-term work.

The King of "Un" is in our corner. Not only that, but He desires a personal relationship with us. A relationship where we can go to Him with our fitness struggles and He will listen. A relationship where we can present our frustrations and He hears us. A relationship where we can ask for strength to overcome and He strengthens us. The King of "Un," the King over all, wants us to approach His throne of grace. When we give him our everything, He will supply our needs.

Unbelievable.

Daily Spiritual Exercise: Memorize a favorite Scripture.
There are many "un" words used to describe God. Pick one of your favorites found in Scripture (that you don't currently have memorized) and commit it to memory.

A good technique for memorizing Scripture is to read the verse ten times in a row. Be sure to cite the book, chapter, and verse each time. Then, close your eyes and say the verse ten times in a row. Do that every day for a week and you have the verse written on the tablet of your heart.

This method is especially helpful for learning long passages. Let's say you have 12 verses to memorize. Day 1, you read verse one ten times, then say it from memory ten times. On Day 2, recite verse one from memory. Then, read verse two ten times. Afterward, say verse two ten times from memory. Day 3, recall verses one and two from memory, and move on to verse three. Repeat this until you know all 12 verses.

David tells us:

> *"I will meditate on your precepts and fix my eyes on your ways."*
> *−Psalm 119:15 (ESV)*

The better we know the Word, the better we can know the King. There's no better way to know the word than to memorize it.

Week 4 Day 1 | *The King of "Un": Undone*

Undone. It's one of my favorite words to describe the results of Christ's death on the cross. What was done, our sin, is gone. As 1 John says, our sins have been taken away:

> *"But you know that he appeared so that he might take away our sins. And in him is no sin."–3:5 (NIV)*

Where our sins were, they are no more, because in Him there is no sin. What we did has been . . . undone.

What's interesting is that in light of the cross, "undone" completes the work Jesus came to do. He resolves the mess we left unresolved.

What's also noteworthy is that "undone" is actually the antithesis of another meaning of the word, that of being unfinished. However, Jesus finished His Father's task for Him on Earth, and in so doing, He made us complete, marked us as His, and not lacking any good thing.

When I think of "undone," I inadvertently think of a knotted shoe-lace. Ever had a knot so tight that you thought it would never come out? Maybe you could pick at it with a fork. Perhaps you had to cut it out with scissors. Or you thought you could eventually untie it, but you'd need two pairs of pliers and some serious fortitude. Regardless of your approach, one thing was going to happen, maybe two. First, *you* were going to be the one to get the knot out. *You* would be responsible for fixing it. Secondly, there would be a reasonable chance your laces would be ruined in the process. Both propositions were unpleasant, frustration would ensue, and defeat would soon follow.

That is our sin. However, in the infinite beauty of the cross, the knots of sin in our lives that get twisted and snarled are unraveled. Undone.

In His perfect sovereignty, Jesus tied Himself to a tree. In so doing, the bonds of death were untied. Undone.

There's no need for us to pick at our knots with a fork. No need to cut them out with scissors or tug at them with pliers. He knew we were helpless on our own, so He undid the bonds for us.

The beauty doesn't stop there. If you look at a shoelace, there's no real evidence that it was ever previously knotted. It just looks like a shoelace. That's how we appear to the Father—unblemished, without evidence of sin, without blame. Our knots are no more and we are freed to live in a way that brings Him glory.

It sure is easy to get stuck in the past. It's easy to focus on our failures, dwell on the negative, focus on our knots. Perhaps it's even easier to try to fix it all ourselves. The thing is . . . we can't.

It's easier to see more of what we've done wrong with fitness than what we've done right, but God doesn't see it like that. He sees opportunity to do what we couldn't do on our own. If we present our struggles to the Lord, He can replace them with victory.

What issues are holding you back with your fitness? Is it the eating, be it too much of the wrong things or too little of the right ones? Is it the pride of making your temple your god rather than letting Him be the God of your temple? Is lethargy weighing you down? Or is there just an ongoing battle with who is on the throne of your heart? Who you go to as your source of strength and comfort?

We need to present these entanglements to our loving Father daily, hourly, sometimes even moment by moment. He and only He has the power to conquer our sin. To equip us for victory. To undo what's been done.

Prayer
Father, thank You for undoing what I could not undo on my own. Will You forgive me when I struggle because I'm trying to operate out of my own strength? Please help me to stay centered on the cross. You haven't just won the war; You can win the battles along the way. Amen.

Meditation

There's nothing I've done that can't be undone by You!

Daily Spiritual Exercise

Memorize a favorite Bible passage reflecting God's ability to undo our mess. One of my favorites is 2 Corinthians 5:21:

> *"God made him who had no sin to be sin for us, so that in him we might become the righteousness of God." (NIV)*

Whatever verse you choose, remember that the purpose of memorizing Scripture is to believe what it is saying. So believe it!

Week 4 Day 2 | *The King of "Un": Unconventional*

Have you ever stopped to consider how unconventional our God is? I don't mean in a quirky or eccentric way. I mean in the sense that He conforms to no rule or precedent that I know. Any preconceptions we may have of who God is are quickly shattered when we get to know His character.

Take some of the most famous champions found in Scripture and you'll quickly see that they are deeply flawed beings. They are laden with insecurities and doubt, mired in sin and failure. They are certainly not the kind of people you or I would likely choose to help build the kingdom.

Take some of the most prominent stories in the Bible. They unfold in ways that, on the surface, leave you scratching your head. A giant boat, every kind of land animal on the planet, and a worldwide flood. The dude who gets swallowed by a fish and lives there for a few days. The walls of an enemy city fall, but only after they were encircled for a week; oh, and priests blow in some rams' horns. One unorthodox story after another.

Then, in the greatest act of love the world has ever known, perfect Jesus comes down to a very imperfect Earth. He chooses not a palace for his birth, but a stable. He chooses not a king for a Dad, but a carpenter. He chooses not to be served, but to serve. He forgoes comfort, ease, and pleasure in exchange for a physically, emotionally, and spiritually excruciating death.

There is nothing conventional about Jesus Christ.

Every time we go on a road trip, a barrage of questions is hurled at us from the backseat. Like grenades from the trenches, they're coming at us: "How much longer?" "Why are we going this way?" "Why can't we eat now?" "Do we really need to stop for gas?" "Can we stop for the potty?" "Do you know where you're going?" That's just as we're pulling out of the neighborhood!

While such questions can be frustrating, from a kids' standpoint they're understandable. They really don't know the way. They don't know how to get from here to there. They don't know when it's best to do what.

They're on a road trip and have questions that they think deserve answers. They don't know the whole plan.

Our God knows the full story, though. He knows the entire script.

When Noah spent year after year building that colossal ark, he probably had a question with every pound of his hammer . . . God knew the script. As Jonah was sliding down the gullet of a big fish thinking it was the end . . . God knew the script. When the rooster crowed for the third time and a guilt-ridden Peter looked into the eyes of Christ . . . God knew the script.

Given that God does things differently, have you considered that He has plans for your fitness struggles? You would probably write your story free of pain or conflict, and reaching every fitness goal you set. God, however, deals in the dilemmas, frustrations, and failures. He's a master at snatching triumph out of the jaws of defeat.

If you're open to God's leading, He can and will bring glory to Himself out of your fitness disappointments. That's the exciting thing! While we might not know the full script, the road trip, we do know the ending. The victory is already won. For that very reason we must trust the author and finisher of our faith:

> *"For my thoughts are not your thoughts, neither are your ways my ways,' declares the Lord."—Isaiah 55:8 (NIV)*

His ways are not our ways; they're higher. His thoughts are not our thoughts; they're higher. Therefore, could it be that God has a plan for your fitness that you had not envisioned?

When you come to accept that He knows what we don't and He does what we wouldn't, "conventional" quickly becomes overrated.

Prayer

Father, thank You for not leaving the script up to me. Will You please forgive me when I think I know best? Please give me greater faith to trust You in all things. May my fitness be used, in whatever way, for your glory. Amen.

Meditation

Your ways are not my ways . . . please align my thoughts to yours.

Daily Spiritual Exercise

Memorize a favorite Bible passage reflecting the unconventional nature of God's character. Isaiah 55:8 is a great option, as is Psalm 89:6–8, Exodus 8:10, and Isaiah 40:18. Whichever passage you choose, the point is to keep it at the forefront of your mind when things don't go the way you think they should.

Week 4 Day 3 | *The King of "Un": Unfailing*

Our world is filled with one failure after another. The news is a continual montage of broken people in broken stories living broken lives in this broken world. It's like watching a cash register spit out a never-ending receipt. Political scandals, celebrity meltdowns, corporate greed, economic ruin, personal destruction, environmental disasters, and civil unrest. If your heart is left unguarded, current events can become depressing quite quickly. Though if it's any consolation, since the fall of man it's always been this way.

A quick stroll through Scripture also reads like the news, with one sad story after another. Each one exemplifies how men fail when they aren't reliant on God as their source of strength, comfort, and contentment. Adam and Eve get greedy and disobey. Cain gets jealous and murders his brother. Noah gets drunk. Moses disobeys. Abraham deceives. Jacob dishonors his father and cheats his brother. David lusts, commits adultery, and kills. Solomon disobeys, intermarries, and worships foreign gods. Judas betrays Christ, and Peter denies Him. Failure abounds, much as it does today.

Yet, since the beginning of time, God knew that apart from Him, we would mess things up. This also means that He proceeded knowing how to use our sin for His glory.

Take David, for example. When God was creating David, God knew he would fail Him in a big way. God still used David. To this day, David is one of the most powerful, influential writers in the Bible. His failure was used by God for our good.

No wonder that when you look at the Psalms that David wrote, you see how he described God's love as "unfailing":

> *"Let your face shine on your servant; save me in your unfailing love."*—Psalm 31:16 (NIV)

David knew probably better than anyone the restorative, empowering, satisfying, and sanctifying love of God . . . His unfailing love.

In fact, the word "unfailing" appears 33 times in the Book of Psalms. What's interesting is that each writer is referring to God and follows unfailing with the word "love." Unfailing love.

When God was creating Peter, He knew Peter would succumb to fear and deny Jesus all three times. However, God used that failure to perfect Peter's faith to the point where it led to his own crucifixion. This ultimately united Peter with Christ and left an inspiring example for the church. Unfailing love.

Before God created Judas, He knew Judas would turn on Jesus for a bag of silver. Yet He used that failure for His purpose, which ultimately led to our salvation on the cross. Unfailing love.

Even before He created you and me, God knew we would fail Him. However, He loved us so much that He created us anyway, knowing He could use us for His glory no matter what.

Most people don't win at fitness the first time they try. They may not even win the second or third time. We fail to start when we should. We fail to stay the course. We fail to align our motives to His. We fail to keep Him on His rightful place in our hearts. We fail to rely on His strength. We fail to include Him in the journey.

God has a plan for all that failure and that's to use it for His purposes. Since the beginning of time, God has planned to use His unfailing love to restore a fallen world back to perfection. A love that removes every blemish, wipes clean every mistake, and heals every wound.

This isn't, however, an excuse to keep failing. It's an encouragement to know our efforts can be recycled for His purposes. It's an assurance to know that with God, nothing is wasted. It's a liberation to know that He re-engineers our failure for our freedom. It's a declaration that should embolden you to triumph knowing that His love has not . . . will not . . . and cannot . . . fail.

No matter what our history is with fitness, God has erased our failings. If we present those to Him, He can bring victory.

Prayer

Father, thank You for taking failure and making something good out of it. Will You forgive me when I'm complacent about my sin and take advantage of Your grace? Please help me to be victorious in who You created me to be. Amen.

Meditation

Your unfailing love gives me peace and victory.

Daily Spiritual Exercise

Memorize a favorite Bible passage reflecting the unfailing love of God, such as Psalm 31:16. Let whatever verse you choose be a reminder that by His unfailing love, we are saved. His love has overcome our failure, and by it He deserves all glory and honor.

Week 4 Day 4 | *The King of "Un": Unparalleled*

I am a sucker for nature shows. The breadth of design of animals is staggering, and it doesn't stop with their looks. Their instincts, abilities, and roles in keeping Earth's grand design moving are incredible.

Plants are no less amazing. All shades and shapes play a part in an ever-moving masterpiece of beauty and function. To add to the bewilderment, we are nowhere near done discovering new species. According to the World Wildlife Fund, 441 new species of plants and animals were discovered in a remote part of the Amazon rain forest between 2010 and 2013. Think of that: 441 undiscovered species in just one small, faraway part of the planet! Furthermore, the earth is nearly three-fourths covered in water. Just think about how much we don't yet know about marine life.

The weather is equally fascinating. It has a purpose specific to each region and a life-sustaining contribution to the world at large. Beyond its constant change and provision, it brings matchless beauty. What can compare to the distant splendor of a sunset? Or a coming storm? Sunrays poking holes in cloud cover? Have you ever seen images of a snowflake under a microscope? Not only is its structure utterly complex, but it's also completely unique. Not one snowflake that has fallen or will ever fall is exactly like any other snowflake that has fallen or will ever fall.

When we look up even higher, we see the moons, planets, stars, constellations, and galaxies that go on without end. Year after year, scientists discover new heavenly bodies. The universe is ever expanding and, for the Christian, ever expanding our view of our Creator.

Perhaps the greatest benefit of studying nature is the most paradoxical. The more we understand its design, the more we get to know its Creator. Yet the more we understand nature, the more we realize the vast difference between God's ability and ours. We would do well to succumb to the futility of trying to fully comprehend the power of the One who created it. The mind just can't conceive.

"Who is like the Lord?" We read phrases like this in the Bible and we rightfully think of God's mighty strength and His glory. Knowing He handcrafted every animal, hand-painted every plant, hand-placed every star . . . how can we not be in awe of His works?

In Psalm 89, we read of God's uniqueness. Yet His uniqueness isn't limited to His power. His faithfulness is also unique . . . and deserves greater awe still:

> *"The heavens praise your wonders, Lord, your faithfulness too, in the assembly of the holy ones. For who in the skies above can compare with the Lord? Who is like the Lord among the heavenly beings? In the council of the holy ones God is greatly feared; he is more awesome than all who surround him. Who is like you, Lord God Almighty? You, Lord, are mighty, and your faithfulness surrounds you."—verses 5–8 (NIV)*

In fact, "faithful" or "faithfulness" appears 10 times throughout Psalm 89 alone. Relating itself to His power, His provision, and His promises, it's like the lines our imaginations draw between stars in constellations.

The scope of power of our Creator-Father has been matched by the faithfulness He has established along with it. It knows no bounds. It is only rational when looking through the lens of love, the same lens through which He looks at us. After all, He sent His Son to save us. His Son sits to the right of His throne up on high, where all that has ever been was conceived. Jesus came down here as the ultimate demonstration of love and faithfulness. When His son returned to His rightful place, in another act of love and faithfulness, God then sent His Holy Spirit. He comes to live in us, love through us, and live out His purposes for us.

There is nothing God can't do. His faithfulness is without measure. Therefore, the only logical response is for us to trust He will continue being who He has always been. The God of all creation has said He will be with us always. He has proven Himself to be forever unequaled in power and faithfulness. We would be wise to rely on the truth of who He is to empower us throughout this fitness journey. He is there to supply our every need when we are struggling with making our fitness a priority. God is there to keep us encouraged when we start to experience some success in our fitness. He's there to keep us focused on Him during our fitness triumphs, that He might receive the glory. He . . . is . . . there.

That, in part, is why there is no one like our Lord. There are none more faithful than He. If we truly trust in His leading and loyalty, the Lord will not disappoint.

So, go on and be in awe. Be amazed at the work of His fingers, but be further amazed at the work of His unparalleled faithfulness.

Prayer
Father, thank You that there truly are none like You. Will You forgive me when I look elsewhere for help from where help can't come? Please guide me to stay focused on You and Your faithfulness. Amen.

Meditation
Your faithfulness is unparalleled.

Daily Spiritual Exercise
Memorize a favorite verse that characterizes God's unparalleled faithfulness, such as Psalm 89:8. Truly, there is no one as powerful, as glorious, or as faithful as the Lord of all creation.

Week 4 Day 5 | *The King of "Un": Unchanging*

The world's pace of change is both exciting and infuriating. It's accelerating so fast that the consequences oftentimes bring optimism and dejection in equal parts. For every advancement in medicine that gives us hope, we uncover a new kind of infection that makes us panic. Technology is getting faster, smarter, and smaller, while also making last year's "next big thing" nearly obsolete. Geopolitically, a new democratic republic may be created in one part of the world while a former republic is overtaken in another.

This pace-of-change phenomenon happens with our fitness too. We learn new things about the body and then realize we've been doing it wrong all this time. Remember the low-fat/high-carb craze of the '90s? The dizzying array of innovations, discoveries, and all their implications bombard us from every angle, all the time. To make matters worse, change is showing no signs of slowing down.

However, our Father changes all that for us, by remaining unchanged Himself. Imagine . . . we have access to the One who spun the world into place, shifts the tides, and switches the seasons. Yet He Himself remains immovable, resolute, and steadfast. We see this unchanging nature of His character displayed throughout Scripture.

Men change their minds on a whim, but what God says He'll do, He does (Numbers 23:19). *His intentions are unchanging.*

Our words are in the air for but a moment, but His Word is eternal (Psalm 119:89); it endures forever (Isaiah 40:8). *His Word is unchanging.*

Our energy and ability are finite, but He is everlasting, does not grow tired, and does not grow weary (Isaiah 40:28). *His strength is unchanging.*

Leaders rise and rulers fall, but He has ruled forever (Psalm 55:19). *His reign is unchanging.*

Our lives are but a breath, but He has always been (Psalm 102:27). *His years are unchanging.*

Our loyalties waver and our fortitude fails, but His faithfulness continues throughout all generations (Psalm 119:90). *His faithfulness is unchanging.*

What man does, doesn't last. Whatever God does is complete, lacking nothing, lasting forever (Ecclesiastes 3:14). *His works are unchanging.*

The purposes for which man lives fluctuate with the times, but not the Lord's (Malachi 3:6). *His purposes are unchanging.*

Man gives reluctantly, incompletely, and with improper motives, but God gives willingly, lovingly, and perfectly (James 1:17). *His generosity is unchanging.*

Whereas we have unkept promises, it's impossible for God to lie (Hebrews 6:17–18). *His promises are unchanging.*

Our pastors have temporary positions, but God's Son has a position that will last forever (Hebrews 7:24). *His Son's priesthood is unchanging.*

Where theologies rise, religions fall, and movements fail, God's Son is the same yesterday, today, and tomorrow (Hebrews 13:8). *His Son is unchanging.*

While we will betray, fall short, and lose faith, God's Son remains ever faithful (2 Timothy 2:13). *His Son's faithfulness is unchanging.*

There is great comfort to be found in His consistent trustworthiness. While God is unchanging in who He is, He can change you. In fact, because He is unchanging, He is also the only logical and deserving foundation to power change in you. God can help us with the physical changes we're seeking, assuming we're seeking Him to first change our hearts. To be molding them. To be shaping them. To be making them more like His. All the changes we want on the outside won't honor Him in the least, if we're not changed on the inside.

If the pace of life during this fitness journey is stressing you, take heart. If the thought of change scares you or the speed at which the world is spinning unsettles you . . . pause. Exhale. Take in a little air, then breathe out again, deeper this time. Relax your shoulders. Untense your neck. Clear your mind. Stop for a second, or a minute.

Now ask yourself, "Who is in control?"

If God is in control and if He is unchanging, we can trust him to do what only he can do perfectly—empower us.

Then remind yourself, the more things change, the more God stays the same.

Prayer

Father, thank You for Your steadfastness. Will You forgive me when I seek the wrong kind of change? Please help me always rely on who You are and have always been. Amen.

Meditation

You are unchanging.

Daily Spiritual Exercise

Memorize a favorite verse or passage reflecting God's unchanging nature. I'm fond of Numbers 23:19 and the bluntness used to quickly put God's character in perspective. Then be sure to start believing in your heart what you're putting in your head . . . God has not, does not, and will not change.

Week 4 Day 6 | *The King of "Un": Unrelenting*

If something is said to be "unrelenting," it usually sounds like a bad thing. Unrelenting is most often used to describe a noun that's negative: pain, sadness, cruelty, adversity, destruction, struggle, or poverty. Truly, the world is filled with an endless onslaught of bad news. However, the Word of God is filled with story after story of good news. That good is always rooted in the same thing: God's unrelenting love.

In the beginning, God loved mankind enough to create a perfect Earth for him. He loved man enough to create him in His own image. God loved man enough to put him in charge of this perfect earth. He loved man enough to create woman. He loved them enough to bless them with all He had created. That's just in Genesis 1.

Fast-forward and we see that when man needed leaders, God loved mankind enough to provide them. There's Noah, Abraham, Joseph, Moses, David, Solomon, Daniel, John the Baptist, Peter, and Paul, to name a few.

Whenever mankind needed escape, provision, protection, or victory, God loved them enough to provide it:

- The ark
- Manna from heaven
- Parting of the Red Sea
- Walls of Jericho
- Defeat of Amalekites
- Defeat of the Midianites
- Defeat of Ai
- Joseph in the well
- The death of Goliath
- Safety from King Saul
- Daniel and the lion's den
- Shadrach, Meshach, and Abednego in the furnace
- Rahab and the spies

When mankind needed godly examples to follow, God loved them enough to provide them. We see this with Job, Joseph, Ruth, Moses, David, Daniel, Elijah, Peter, Paul, Stephen, John the Baptist, and Mary and Joseph.

When mankind had physical needs, God loved them enough to send Jesus to take care of them. Lepers healed. Sight is restored. The lame walk. Hemorrhaging is stopped. Deaf ears are opened. Water is turned into wine. Bread and fish are multiplied. Demons are cast out. Storms are calmed. Ears are attached. Lazarus, the widow's son, and Jairus's daughter are all resurrected.

Most importantly, when mankind had a spiritual need, God loved him so much that He sent Jesus, who lived a perfect life and died an undeserved death. Why? To bury all our sins and to be raised to life again. He is forever united with His heavenly Father and made forever available to His children.

Throughout Scripture, we have one example after another of good news—God demonstrating a love that met the physical, emotional, and spiritual needs of His children. I bet that if you look at your life, you could find example after example of Him doing the same. I certainly can.

I was born healthy into a wonderful Christian family, in a safe environment. I attended Bible-teaching churches, went to a Christian school, and had fantastic friends. While I grew up chubby and was teased for it, God used it to shape my passions and perspective.

In my mid-20s, I married a God-fearing woman. She helped open my eyes, challenge me, mature me, and grow me in my walk with Him. We had a lot of debt. Yet God used that to help teach us wise financial stewardship, while also providing career advancement in the process.

Later on, I was unfairly fired from a position with a nonprofit organization. God used that too, opening a position at a small company that gave me many great opportunities for development. He did that, while also orchestrating a mentorship with a man who spoke a lot of truth into my life.

Ten years and three more kids later, I get to teach body stewardship principles for a living. I've left out some of the hardships and disappointments I've experienced. However, I know for a fact God used them and is continuing to use them to mold my faith. I'm confident also that there are countless times He's protected me from things I don't know about: accidents, relationships, bad business opportunities, and sicknesses.

The point is that I know He is working at all times in all things. I've seen it in Scripture. I've seen it in the lives of others. I've certainly seen it in my own life. It's just part of his nature . . . He is unrelenting.

David certainly understood that wherever we are, God is there, chasing our hearts and minds without ceasing. In fact, the first 12 verses of Psalm 139 detail just how present and determined God is.

Verses 7 and 10 summarize it well:

> *"I can never escape from your Spirit! I can never get away from your presence!" "Even there your hand will guide me, and your strength will support me." (NLT)*

If that's the case, if our King has always been unrelenting, why would He stop now? He wouldn't! He will continue to be unrelenting in the pursuit of our hearts. Even now, maybe especially now, He seeks our hearts as we learn how to better care for our bodies.

> *". . . neither our fears for today nor our worries about tomorrow— not even the powers of hell can separate us from God's love. No power in the sky above or in the earth below—indeed, nothing in all creation will ever be able to separate us from the love of God that is revealed in Christ Jesus our Lord."—Romans 8:38b–39 (NLT)*

Our fears or worries can't stop Him. Space and time don't deter Him. Whether up high or down low, in our minds or on our hearts, He won't slow down. Nothing of any kind anywhere can impede the unrelenting pursuit of our King.

Our Father never stops pursuing us, pouring out Himself on us, and providing for us. Therefore, we can be emboldened and empowered by His presence in us. Out of that same strength, with unwavering determination we can pursue not only our fitness but more importantly our faith. Then we, too, can be characterized by the word "unrelenting." That sounds like a good thing to me.

Prayer

Father, thank You for pursuing me with such wild abandonment. Will You forgive me when I pursue the wrong things or even the right things but for the wrong reasons? Please help me to always be pursuing Your heart. Amen.

Meditation

Your love is unrelenting.

Daily Spiritual Exercise

Memorize a favorite Scripture passage demonstrating God's unrelenting love. Romans 8:38–39 might be a good place to start. Know He is unrelenting, and if He is in you, then you can be unrelenting too.

Week 4 Day 7 | *The King of "Un": Unending*

In the Toy Story trilogy, beloved spaceman Buzz Lightyear likes to belt out his trademark mantra, "To infinity and beyond." Now we love Pixar movies and, admittedly, Buzz's catchphrase sounds great, but it's kind of nonsensical, really. Infinity is hard enough to get your mind around. How can you go past it?

It's understandable that we struggle with the notions of timelessness or eternity. After all, our entire lives are bookended. We have only known phases, each varied in length, but all with definite starts and stops. Within those seasons, we have a limited quantity of resources to see us through: time, money, energy, interest, ability, and so forth. To include God and the endless supply of all that He is, it's foreign to all we have ever known. To make things harder to grasp, there was never a starting point to "The" Supply to begin with . . . He just always was.

The Bible assures us that where our King is concerned, there is no start or finish. Our finite minds can trust our infinite God. The sooner we live our lives through the lens of eternity, the more fulfilling it will be. To help us permanently adopt that outlook, we need to "press pause" on our intellects for a moment. Then, we must look to the Word for reminders that God is not constrained by space or time.

First of all, as God, He is unending. Psalm 90:2 says, "Before the mountains were born or you brought forth the whole world, from everlasting to everlasting you are God."

As Lord, He is eternal. Habakkuk 1:12 says, "Lord, are you not from everlasting? My God, my Holy One, you will never die."

As Father, He is everlasting. We are reminded this every Christmas when we sing Handel's "Messiah". Taken from Isaiah 9:6, we sing, "And he will be called Wonderful Counselor, Mighty God, Everlasting Father, Prince of Peace."

Or, as Revelation 1:8 so aptly summarizes, the Lord God "who is, and who was, and who is to come, the Almighty."

It would then follow suit that our eternal Rock (Isaiah 26:4), our eternal King (Jeremiah 10:10), the Alpha and Omega, would operate in the realm of the unending. We see that played out as His righteous laws (Psalm 119:160), His Word (Psalm119:89), His power (Romans 1:20), and His purpose (Ephesians 3:11) are all eternal.

Out of that everlasting power and purpose, He does things that only an eternal God could do. He makes countless descendants (Jeremiah 33:22), everlasting covenants (Ezekiel 37:26), and everlasting signs (Isaiah 55:13). Out of His everlasting love (Jeremiah 31:3), He gives everlasting names (Isaiah 56:5) and crowns heads with everlasting joy (Isaiah 35:10). He guides with an everlasting light (Isaiah 60:19–20) from an everlasting kingdom (Psalm 145:13) and dominion (Daniel 7:14).

All of this sounds great, but even still, it can feel a little distant—that is, until we look at how His unending nature applies to us personally. We are told that any persecution we experience for our faith is outweighed by the eternal glory we will achieve (2 Corinthians 4:17). Psalm 16:11 says that He can fill us with the joy of His presence, with eternal pleasures at His right hand. Out of His presence, by grace, He gives us eternal encouragement (2 Thessalonians 2:16). We can live by His eternal Spirit (Hebrews 9:14) so that we may receive the eternal inheritance (Hebrews 9:15) in an eternal house (2 Corinthians 5:1) for our eternal lives:

> *"For God so loved the world that he gave his one and only Son, that whoever believes in him shall not perish but have eternal life."—John 3:16 (NIV)*

Suddenly, when we see how His everlasting nature applies to our eternal lives, we feel invigorated for our earthly lives. We should feel empowered for all that we face now, including our fitness. God is there to help us. He does not grow tired or weary (Isaiah 40:28), and His love for us is from everlasting to everlasting (Psalm 103:17). Out of that love, He can help us bring glory back to Him, even with our health. In fact, He can do far more than that:

> *"Now to him who is able to do immeasurably more than all we ask or imagine, according to his power that is at work within us . . ."*
> *—Ephesians 3:20 (NIV)*

Wow! "According to His power that is at work within us." Daily surrender. Repeat humbling. Spirit living. Therefore, we need to consistently rely on His power in us to live out our faith. This, in turn, can also help us live out our quest for fitness.

God can do what again? "Immeasurably more." So much more that it can't be quantified or qualified. It can't be captured, contained, or counted. It's more than we can think to ask to begin with. It's more than we can imagine we could experience in the end.

If there is no end to our God or His abilities or His nature, there is no end to how much He can empower our fitness.

What the result of His involvement with your fitness will ultimately look like, I can't say. What it looks like for your faith, I can't imagine.

I do know that the more we experience His power in us, the more we can get a glimpse of its unending nature.

The greater the glimpse, the better we understand that He and only He could ever truly encompass . . . infinity and beyond.

Prayer
Father, thank You that You are not limited by what I can ask or imagine. Will You forgive me when I operate out of my own power to fill a role only You can fill? Please help me to always rely on the endless supply of your nature.

Meditation
You are endless in grace, glory, love, and provision.

Daily Spiritual Exercise
Memorize a Bible passage that portrays the endless nature of God's love, glory, provision, or power. Certainly New Testament favorite Ephesians 3:20–21 captures the sentiment. As always, make it your ambition to own in your heart what you're committing to your mind.

The Holy Spirit is easily the most misunderstood member of the Trinity. First of all, we tend to think of Him in terms of the New Testament only. Genesis suggests a different story. Some believe that in Genesis 1:1, the Hebrew word "elohiym" is used as the plural form of God, implying the three-in-one Godhead. We also see in verse two, when "the Spirit of God" moved over the waters:

> "In the beginning God created the heavens and the earth. Now the earth was formless and empty, darkness was over the surface of the deep, and the Spirit of God was hovering over the waters."
> —Genesis 1:1–2 (NIV)

Furthermore, in verse 26, God says, "Let us make man in our image, in our likeness…" all referring to multiple beings, and all in the first chapter of the first book of the Bible.

Throughout the Old Testament, the Holy Spirit is referenced. We see the "Spirit of God" at work regenerating faith (Ezekiel 11 and 36). We see Him "coming upon" God's people (Joshua, David, and even Saul). In Exodus 31, He gifts people with special talents, as in the case of Bezalel. As you can see, the Holy Spirit is certainly not confined to the New Testament.

Secondly, the Holy Spirit often seems impersonal to us. For starters, "holy" isn't something we relate to because we are so far from holiness on our own. As if that's not enough, a "spirit" sounds so mystical as we go about living in our physical world. It's no wonder the Holy Spirit seems hard to relate to or understand.

It's critical to our Christian walk that we not only understand the Holy Spirit, but get to know Him . . . intimately. Studying His titles is a great place to start: counselor, advocate, life, seal, wisdom, Spirit of sonship and comforter.

When we define these terms, we paint a picture of the person of the Holy Spirit. That's when we put a little skin on Him.

Then, when we start seeing these words in action, playing out in our own lives, the Holy Spirit makes more sense. We start understanding His character, His power, and His purpose for us. Once you understand these concepts, you can't help falling in love with Him.

Daily Spiritual Exercise: Practice "spiritual breathing" throughout the day. Bill Bright, founder of Campus Crusade for Christ, came up with the practice of "spiritual breathing." Spiritual breathing (exhaling the impure and inhaling the pure) is an exercise in faith. It enables you to know and live in God's ongoing love and forgiveness. Here's how Campus Crusade explains it:

Exhale: Confess your sin. Agree with God concerning your sin and thank Him for His forgiveness of it, according to 1 John 1:9 and Hebrews 10:1–25. Confession involves repentance: a change in attitude and action.

Inhale: Surrender the control of your life to Christ, and appropriate (receive) the fullness of the Holy Spirit by faith. Trust that He now directs and empowers you according to the command of Ephesians 5:18 and the promise of 1 John 5:14–15.

As you go about your day, train yourself in this practice. Spiritual breathing is a wonderful tool for staying in constant communion with our Father and living by the Holy Spirit. It's also very effective in defending against going to the wrong sources for renewal, such as food or lethargy.

Reaching for the Lord first is evidence of the Holy Spirit working in you. The more He works, the more you get to know Him. And the more you get to know Him, the more you benefit and the more the Lord is glorified.

Week 5 Day 1 | *Names for the Holy Spirit: Counselor*

Of the many names given to the Holy Spirit, "counselor" probably has the least pizazz, on the surface anyway. Maybe the term harkens images of being back in school, meeting with a well-intentioned academic counselor—some poor soul tasked with helping you make life-changing decisions based on 10-minute meetings and the scan of a report card. Or maybe thoughts of marriage counseling come to mind. Seeking help on serious issues causing a divide between you and your spouse, while productive, is hardly thrilling. Or perhaps you remember the camp counselor who put a halt on your nightly water balloon excursions. No matter how you look at it, most people wouldn't get too excited about meeting with a counselor of any kind.

However, the Holy Spirit is unlike any other counselor.

First of all, the Holy Spirit is perfect. Therefore, He gives only perfect counsel. Perfect guidance.

Also, the role of Counselor is not merely to guide us:

> *"But the Counselor, the Holy Spirit, whom the Father will send in my name, he will teach you all things, and bring to your remembrance all that I have said to you."—John 14:26 (RSV)*

Jesus says "he will teach you . . . ," so our role as His children is to hold on to His teaching and follow it. Only then is His teaching productive.

Unlike in school when we are taught something but soon forget, the Holy Spirit is there to remind us of what we have learned. Jesus says the Holy Spirit will ". . . bring to your remembrance all that I have said to you."

Just imagine! The Holy Spirit is in our hearts to guide us, teach us, and continually point us back to Jesus and God the Father. Suddenly, having access to the only perfect Counselor gets quite exciting.

"Counselor," unlike other descriptions of the Holy Spirit, requires effort from us for the term to be beneficial in our lives. There is a difference between knowing the right thing to do and doing the right thing.

Knowing just isn't enough.

If we want to benefit from the Counselor and if we want to glorify the Father, we must listen *and* we must follow His counsel . . . His perfect counsel.

We see this with our fitness almost on a daily basis. We need to go to bed earlier, but do we? We need to start working out, but we put it off another week. We know we should try to incorporate more produce into our diets, but we stick with vending machines.

Or maybe you're on the opposite end of the spectrum. Maybe you need to make exercise less of a priority. It's teetering on the edge of becoming a small "g" god. Can you ever really strike a balance without feeling guilty about missing a day in the gym?

Our Counselor helps us, guides us, reminds us, and teaches us. He does this, in part, by directing our hearts and minds back to God, both when we fail and succeed.

One of the neat things about our Counselor is that He is not limited to only teaching and guiding us. He can empower us to both listen and follow through because He's just that big. He's just that powerful. He's just that perfect.

Prayer
Father, thank You for giving us your Spirit, the Counselor. Will You forgive me when You direct my heart and I choose to ignore it? Please continually remind me to rely solely on the power of your Holy Spirit to follow through. Amen.

Meditation
The Holy Spirit both directs my heart and empowers it.

Daily Spiritual Exercise
Practice "spiritual breathing" throughout the day. As you do, ask the Lord to give you a discerning heart, one able to tune in to the counsel of the Holy Spirit. Ask also for the strength to follow His leading and He will fully equip you for every good work, empowering you on to its completion.

Week 5 Day 2 | *Names for the Holy Spirit: Spirit of Life*

Have you ever heard of people being described as "full of life"? They have so much zeal for whatever it is they're doing and they seem to like to do everything. No interest is off-limits. They pour themselves into whatever it is, all the way, often times without considering the consequences.

If I were asked to describe our nine-year-old daughter, Myla, I would say she is full of life. She has boundless energy, being up early and with plenty in her tank at the end of the day when Mom and Dad are tired. Whatever she does, she likes to *really* do it. If she's playing with her dolls, there's no decoration she won't attempt to make. During gymnastics, she soaks in the instruction but also giggles with friends. When competition rolls around, she is focused, devastated when she doesn't bring home a medal, and delighted when she does.

Myla is a strong student who frets over the occasional wrong answer. She's also frequently the impetus for the silly in the house: making faces, telling jokes, directing nonsensical "plays," orchestrating games, dancing to goofy songs, and laughing at her own antics. Just the other day, she was excited to create a multipage chore chart. Her color-coded masterpiece was calendar-based, organized by child, and even included a legend. Like I said, she's enthusiastic for nearly everything.

In order to have such a personality, you have to be wired with an innate sense of freedom. You don't really look at the obstacles in your way. You are either unaware that they exist or you don't care because you feel you can conquer them. While the naiveté that comes with that kind of attitude can cause some heartache, it's an enviable outlook. This inherent life-giving freedom liberates you to pursue your passions without fear of the unknown.

Our faith should be the same way. As Christians, the Holy Spirit lives within us, and the Holy Spirit is the Spirit of Life:

> *"For the law of the Spirit of life in Christ Jesus made me free from the law of sin and of death."—Romans 8:2 (ASV)*

In fact, several times in the Book of Romans, we are told that we have been set free from sin and from death. Christ is the life-giver. As such, our mindset should adopt a permanent sense of liberation, without reservation and without restriction. Then our hearts and minds are like caged animals released into their natural habitats where they belong. When we are focused on Christ, we are free to live as God intended.

With fitness, it's easier to focus on the sacrifices rather than the benefits. When that happens, though, we incarcerate our hearts and minds into cages where life can't be fully experienced. We end up not enjoying the abundance of fruits and vegetables God created for our pleasure. Why? Because we're too busy grumbling about the junk food we can't eat. Or we're preoccupied with dreading a workout rather than appreciating that our bodies were created to do amazing things.

A sacrifice-focused mindset is like staring at the bars on a prison cell. Don't bemoan exercise as a sacrifice. It's a privilege! Don't gloss over the incredible things you can do with the incredible body He has gifted you. Doing so is like fixating on the lock on your cage. Same with lamenting about going to bed early. Or feeling guilty about taking a nap in order to receive the restorative blessing of calm, rest, and sleep.

The Spirit of Life in Christ Jesus saves us from the law of sin and death, giving us eternal life. Could He not also help us live a life characterized by passion, fervor, excitement, and freedom while on Earth? A life centered on the Holy Spirit, bringing us joy even in our fitness? A life where we can enjoy what He has created for us, with us, and in us? A life where an obstacle is merely a nuisance? Where a limitation from one thing is permission to try something else? Where we live as salt and light, and onlookers desire to experience the kind of lives we live?

Myla's middle name is Bliss. When we gave her that name, we obviously had no idea that it would so closely reflect her personality—the way she lives her life.

However, when you and I were born, God knew full well that we could reflect His personality. In order to reflect Him, however, we need the power of the Spirit of Life living in us. Then we can experience the life-giving freedom He brings in all area of our lives, fitness included.

Prayer

Father, thank You for Your Son, and the Spirit of Life who has saved us from sin. Will You forgive me when I'm focused on the wrong things? Please help me to trust in, rely on, and reflect Your life in me. Amen.

Meditation

Holy Spirit, empower me to experience life as you intended.

Daily Spiritual Exercise

Practice "spiritual breathing" throughout the day. As you try to create this habit, pray that you would see it as a gift. Spiritual breathing should not seem or feel like a chore. Ultimately, it's designed to give you more freedom, not less. The more freedom we have in Him, the more we can experience the life He created us to live.

Week 5 Day 3 | *Names for the Holy Spirit: Advocate*

There is a lot to like about an advocate. When someone is fighting for you, speaking on your defense, and pleading for your cause, you feel more assured, more secure.

I used to work as a server in a restaurant. My goal was to give the guests the best experience I could. After all, they were spending their hard-earned money to relax, eat some good food, and enjoy themselves. Sometimes though, things happened beyond my control. A meal was overcooked, someone got the wrong food, or it came out cold. Whatever the case, it was unacceptable. As their server, I would fix it. I would go to the kitchen on my guests' behalf to plead their case and remedy the situation. I was an advocate for my guests.

I also wanted the restaurant represented in a positive light. I wanted the guests to be happy. I wanted them excited to tell their friends about the restaurant and eager to return. I would see to it that incorrect orders were quickly corrected and oftentimes given to them for free. Apologies were also offered. I would send the manager over to ensure the guests were satisfied. I wanted what was best for the restaurant. At that point, I was the restaurant's advocate.

In the Bible (NIV translation), the different uses of the word "advocate" are very instructive. Job uses it when referring to God, as Job tries to set the record straight with his misguided friends. Job 16:9 says, "Even now my witness is in heaven; my advocate is on high." Job is imploring God to vouch for his innocence.

When we move to the New Testament, we see the Apostle John also use the term "advocate." In 1 John 2:1, he writes, "But if anybody does sin, we have an advocate with the Father—Jesus Christ, the Righteous One." Because of Jesus, we are safe with the Father.

In the Gospel of John, Jesus uses "advocate" to describe the Holy Spirit. Jesus, on the other hand, uses the term two different ways. The first is in 14:16, when Jesus says, "And I will ask the Father, and he will give you another advocate to help you and be with you forever…" Now, in addition to Jesus, we have the Holy Spirit working on our behalf.

Then just 10 verses later, the Holy Spirit as an advocate is working, not on our behalf but on Christ's behalf. John 14:26 says, "But the Advocate, the Holy Spirit, whom the Father will send in my name, will teach you all things and will remind you of everything I have said to you."

We see this again in John 15:26, "When the Advocate comes, whom I will send to you from the Father—the Spirit of truth who goes out from the Father—he will testify about me." Then, in John 16:

> *"Unless I go away, the Advocate will not come to you; but if I go, I will send him to you. When he comes, he will prove the world to be in the wrong about sin and righteousness and judgment . . ."*
> *−John 16:7−8 (NIV)*

In each of these instances, the Holy Spirit is advocating for Jesus. He's pleading, defending, and vouching for what the Son of God has accomplished.

This is the great news of our Advocate, the Holy Spirit: He is working both on our behalf and on the Father's!

Whether we are failing with our fitness or having victory, the Holy Spirit is at work. He's at work pleading our struggles before God while lavishing God's love on us. The Holy Spirit is at work in us. He is empowering us to overcome our fitness battles, while reminding us that Jesus has already overcome our sin. The Holy Spirit, the Advocate, is actively working on us to perfect us while working to bring glory back to God the Father.

As I said, there's a lot to like about an advocate, especially ours.

Prayer
Father, thank You for sending your Holy Spirit as an advocate for my behalf and to direct me back to You. Will You forgive me when I take for granted the work the Holy Spirit is doing on my behalf? Please help me always be open to His leading. Amen.

Meditation

The Holy Spirit is working in me, on me, and for me . . . for Him.

Daily Spiritual Exercise

Practice "spiritual breathing" throughout the day. As you do, remember that your spiritual breathing doesn't have to be perfect. The point is to be working on consistently allowing the Holy Spirit to live through you. This, in part, requires honestly and regularly approaching your Father, knowing that the Holy Spirit is interceding on your behalf.

Week 5 Day 4 | *Names for the Holy Spirit: Seal*

Every now and then, my children will attend an event that requires them to pay an admission fee. Once paid, they will receive a stamp on the outside of their hands. The stamp indicates that the admission price has been paid and they are able to attend the event. When they return home, I'll ask them if they had fun. They seem as excited about the stamp on their hands as the event itself. Vowing to never wash their hands again, they want that stamp forever! Of course, over the next few days, the stamp begins to fade and they grow concerned. Their memory of the event is all they have left as proof that they were ever there.

What was it exactly about the stamp that was so special to them? Perhaps they just liked having the artwork temporarily tattooed on their hands where they could see it a lot. I think it was more than that, though. The stamp had significance for them.

First of all, the stamp showed that they had been given authority to come and go to the event. What little kid doesn't want some authority?

Secondly, that authority was genuine and would mean nothing if the stamp had a different design on it. However, the design related to that event. Placed on their hand by someone with even greater authority than they had, the stamp had merit. It was genuine.

The stamp also meant that the children had a sense of belonging. They were a part of a select group that had satisfied the requirement to enter the event. The stamp gave them a special sense of both uniqueness and camaraderie, a small part of a much bigger story. Belonging, genuineness, and authority. No wonder the children were so excited!

You know, as Christians, our admission has been paid. We also have a mark . . . a Seal . . . the Holy Spirit:

> *"When you believed, you were marked in him with a seal, the promised Holy Spirit, who is a deposit guaranteeing our inheritance until the redemption of those who are God's possession—to the praise of his glory."—Ephesians 1:13b–14 (NIV)*

When we become Christians, the Holy Spirit quite literally comes to live inside our bodies (1 Corinthians 6:19). By doing so, the Holy Spirit, among other things, becomes our Seal in the eyes of God. The Holy Spirit has marked our lives. We have the genuine authority to live in heaven where we will belong to our Heavenly Father for all of eternity.

There's more. The Seal doesn't only mark us for life after earth; He empowers us for life on earth. The Seal is the sign that we have access to the storehouse of riches that abound in Christ. It's a mark of what the Holy Spirit can do in our lives, in spite of our lives, through our lives, and for our lives. Notice, it's what "He can do," not what we do. Therefore, we don't have to worry about whether our strength is sustainable as He Himself sustains all things (Hebrews 1:3).

Let's now look at the implications the Seal has for your fitness life. Firstly, He has given you authority to not just enter the storehouse of riches that abound in Christ. You have authority to access them! That's like going into Fort Knox to see the gold and take some home.

The riches found in Christ will help carry out God's will for you as you seek to glorify Him with your health.

Secondly, the Seal is genuine, authentic, and indisputable. You have been marked from on high with a Mark that cannot be undone, overcome, imitated or duplicated. Sometimes we don't think our lives merit success. The Seal says otherwise. The Seal says you have been given freedom for victory because Christ is the victor. He can give you victory with your fitness.

Lastly, the Seal signifies you are a child of God, that you belong to Him. Our Father equips His children (2 Timothy 3:16–17) as He lavishes love and provision in our lives. He endows us with all we need to stay obedient and to bring Him honor . . . in all things.

Unlike the stamp on my children's hands, however, our Seal never fades away. At any time, we can look at our hearts and see Him. Every day lived in His will, by His strength, serves as further proof—a mark that the Holy Spirit is with us even now, working in our lives as a part of a much bigger story.

Prayer

Father, thank You for the authority, genuineness, and belonging that come from the Seal. Will You forgive me when I live or act like someone who has not been sealed with the Holy Spirit? Please help me always rely on the Seal and the gifts that come with Him. Amen.

Meditation

I have been sealed by the perfect Holy Spirit.

Daily Spiritual Exercise

Practice "spiritual breathing" throughout the day. If this becomes difficult and you need help, don't hesitate to ask for it. Remember, the Seal has qualified you to approach the Lord in confidence, to participate in His glory, and to be empowered by Him . . . for you are His!

Week 5 Day 5 | *Names for the Holy Spirit: Spirit of Wisdom*

How would you define "wisdom?" It's certainly more than knowledge, though it requires knowledge. It's also more than experience, though it's most often garnered through experience. Wisdom requires good judgment and the ability to assess the delicate nuances of a situation. It also thinks through the implications of all the options. I would define wisdom this way: the application of experience, knowledge, and judgment to achieve the optimal outcome.

We see men throughout Scripture who were given great wisdom: Bezalel (Exodus 31:3), Joshua (Deuteronomy 34:9), Daniel (Daniel 2:23) and, of course, Solomon. If you remember back in Week 2, we took a close look at Solomon. He made an unlikely choice when God offered to give Solomon whatever he wanted. Solomon chose wisdom—not wealth or women or prestige or power. He was a new leader with a kingship inherited from his father David. Yet out of Solomon's wisdom, he requested more.

The Bible illustrates different kinds of wisdom. There is skill-based wisdom, such as the kind needed for making garments (Exodus 28:3) or metal- working (1 Kings 7:14). There is the kind needed for administering justice (1 Kings 3:28) or for gaining favor (Acts 7:10). There is the kind needed to lead people (2 Chronicles 1:10). There is also the kind needed to withstand the enemy (Luke 21:15). The list goes on.

That's why the Bible urges us to do whatever we can to find wisdom (Proverbs 4:5). The Bible tells us that those who find it are blessed (Proverbs 3:13). For when we have wisdom, we see that it is more valuable than gold (Proverbs 16:16), saves us from the ways of the wicked (Proverbs 2:12), gives nourishment to our bones (Proverbs 3:8), and adds years to our lives (Proverbs 9:11).

Wisdom is not overrated.

Where in life do you find you need wisdom most? Why? What areas in your life would drastically change if you had more wisdom? Is it with your children so that you can rear them in a God-honoring, Christ-centered way? Is it with a dating relationship, so that you marry the "right" person? Do you need wisdom with finding a job where you can be fulfilled in your work? Maybe it's your finances, so you can prepare properly for future needs while giving more to God's work now.

I'm guessing you would also like some wisdom with your fitness. There are countless resources, exercise programs, nutritional supplements, tips, gyms, and websites to navigate. Yet it can be intimidating to know which ones would most likely help you reach your goals. Having some wisdom to discern good from best and what would work most effectively for you would be revolutionary.

Let's not stop there. I want to challenge you to go broader and deeper on your goals for wisdom. For wisdom goes far beyond surviving and even thriving through life's decisions. In fact, Paul gives us the best reason in his letter to the church in Ephesus:

> "I keep asking that the God of our Lord Jesus Christ, the glorious Father, may give you the Spirit of wisdom and revelation, so that you may know him better."–Ephesians 1:17 (NIV)

Did you catch that? He's asking God the Father to give them wisdom for what reason? "So that you may know him better." So you can have an intimate relationship with Him. So you understand His ways and learn better how to walk in them. So your heart can be enlightened to know greater hope. To know the reward you will have in heaven. To know the power you have on Earth (Ephesians 1:18). Knowing the Lord better is the ultimate purpose for our wisdom and should be our first goal in seeking it.

In John Piper's excellent book *Desiring God*, he reminds us that "the chief end of man is to glorify God by enjoying Him forever." If that's the case, then the better we know God, the more we will enjoy Him. The more we enjoy Him, the more we can glorify Him. And glorifying Him is our primary objective of being a good steward of our bodies.

Therefore, we should make every effort to get to know God better. This will require us to rely on the Holy Spirit in us, the Spirit of Wisdom.

Notice a trend? Once again, it's the Holy Spirit working in us that will guide us. When He guides us, God is glorified.

God is eager to give wisdom (James 1:5), so pray for it, including wisdom for your fitness. Then, as you do, expand the purpose for which you're seeking the wisdom you need. Look for ways to understand Him deeper throughout this time. Listen to what the Holy Spirit is trying to tell you. Learn from the lessons He wants to teach you. Know that the wisdom God imparts is there to help you know Him better.

Yes, getting fit is great. However, the degree to which it leads you to a stronger relationship with your Father is far greater.

Prayer
Father, thank You for being generous with your wisdom. Will You forgive when I fail to use it to know you better? Please help me to always keep the greater purpose in mind. Amen.

Meditation
The Holy Spirit is the Spirit of Wisdom.

Daily Spiritual Exercise
Practice "spiritual breathing" throughout the day. As you continually reach out to the Lord, remember to pray for wisdom. Remember, do not pray only for wisdom with your fitness. Pray also that His wisdom will help you know Him better as you're striving to glorify Him with your body.

Week 5 Day 6 | *Names for the Holy Spirit: The Comforter*

From time to time, I like to tackle do-it-yourself (DIY) projects. I've done simple things, such as replace light fixtures, ceiling fans, and plumbing hardware. I've done slightly more complex tasks: building bookshelves, window boxes, and raised garden beds. I've also done more advanced projects, including building a shed and finishing our basement. I'm certainly no pro and I know my limits.

I also know that regardless of the project, at least one factor can determine the rate of progress: the tools. For instance, trying to unscrew faucet hardware with an adjustable wrench is an exercise in busted knuckles and utter frustration . . . not that I'd know. However, if you have a "basin wrench," it takes seconds. Try ripping long, straight sheets of plywood with a reciprocal saw. Not gonna happen. You'll be sanding for days trying to make your edges straight. Do it with a table saw, however, and they're perfect every time.

Even simple things, such as using a rubber mallet rather than a hammer to protect finishes, provide a better end product. Each tool has a purpose specific to the task. If it can complete the job thoroughly and efficiently, it's the right tool. Trust me, the right tool makes all the difference.

Spiritually speaking, however, how easy is it to reach for the wrong tools? A bad workday or stressful moments with the kids has us reaching for pizza or chocolate or both. An argument with our parents results in a mind-numbing escape to the Internet for a couple hours. A bad breakup has us renting sappy love movies. Then, rather than waking up early to exercise, we sleep in, postponing life for just a little while longer. Or perhaps it's the opposite. The rough times we're facing have us obsessed with working out. Soon enough, we are trying to outrun, out-lift, out-bike, out-stretch, and basically outwork our issues. At this point the gym has become nothing more than a hiding place.

Instead of calling out to God, diving into Scripture or singing songs of praise, we do something else. We aren't being still in Him or relying on the Holy Spirit in us. Nope, we try to self-medicate by reaching for the wrong tools in our own form of spiritual DIY. In so doing, the screws break, the wood warps, and we get splinters in our hands. The "project" is a giant mess because the wrong tool falls short every time.

Fortunately, for Christians, our Father specializes in fixing things. He is the God of all comfort (2 Corinthians 1:3–11), who never leaves or forsakes us (Hebrew 13:5), and has given us eternal comfort (2 Thessalonians 2:16–17).

Out of His goodness to us, He sent His Son to die for our salvation. Then He sent His Holy Spirit to minister to us and comfort us until we are united with Him.

You see, the same Greek word used to describe the Holy Spirit as our advocate and counselor, *parakletos*, can also be translated as "helper" or "comforter." How fitting to find, once again, that no single word can adequately describe any one person of the Trinity . . . let alone all three.

Now when we read John 14, we do so in a whole new light:

> *"And I will ask the Father, and he will give you another Helper, to be with you forever,"–verse 16 (ESV)*

A helper sent to comfort us, forever. A comforter who can satisfy us in a way that pizza and chocolate, exercise and sleep, TV, movies and the Internet cannot. Remember, we are notoriously bad tool pickers, and the wrong tools fall short every time.

The Holy Spirit, however, never falls short. As with the right tool in some DIY project, the Holy Spirit's purpose is specific for the task. He can complete it thoroughly and efficiently every time. In DIY, however, the right tool still needs skilled hands to be productive. Not so with the Holy Spirit. He is wholly sufficient on His own. In fact, the more we try to do things on our own, the less effective we are. It's like squirming in quicksand; the harder we try, the faster we sink. That's why spiritual DIY doesn't work. We need more of Him and less of us.

No surprise, God made provisions for our insufficiency too:

"But the Helper, the Holy Spirit, whom the Father will send in my name, he will teach you all things and bring to your remembrance all that I have said to you."—John 14:26 (ESV)

Struggling with your fitness can have you reaching for the wrong tools. Use them and not only will it make little difference, but it's going to hurt. That hurt will have you longing for help.

Stop. Listen to the voice whispering in the quiet of your heart. Hear Him? That is the Helper, the Master Comforter. Sent from the Master Craftsman, He can nurture your soul. He can remind you of all that Jesus, the Master Rabbi, has taught us in the Word.

When you hear the Comforter's voice calling and feel Him working within you, follow in obedience.

You'll quickly see that the Holy Spirit makes all the difference.

Prayer
Father, thank You for sending the Holy Spirit to comfort me. Will You forgive me when I reach for the wrong tools? Please help me to get out of my own way and to allow the Helper to work within me. Amen.

Meditation
You are the Comforter and You give comfort.

Daily Spiritual Exercise
Practice "spiritual breathing" throughout the day. Also, pray for comfort, knowing that the Holy Spirit will direct us back to the Father, reminding us what He has said and done.

Week 5 Day 7 | *Names for the Holy Spirit: Spirit of Sonship*

Our oldest son, Jordan, amazes me. He's smart without trying. He's easy-going and doesn't get rattled very often. He is compliant. Whenever we ask him to do something, He does it, almost always with a great attitude.

Jordan is also a natural communicator. Even at a very young age, he could carry on conversations with adults without any awkwardness. His ability to be at ease when talking to anyone plays into his biggest strength: he's a people person. He loves people, and people love him. He has a charisma that draws people to him and He gets along with most everyone. Since he makes friends so easily, he has a million of them. With all these areas of giftedness, Jordan is among those who could be anything they want to be in life.

I'm very blessed to have a son like Jordan. Now, I call him my son, but, technically, Jordan is not "mine." I married Jordan's mommy when he had begun third grade. I would have loved to have officially adopted Jordan, but it was never an option. I wanted him to have my last name. I wanted him to know that he belonged in the full heritage of my family. Nothing could separate him from that.

I introduce myself as Jordan's "dad," and introduce him to others as my son, rather than "stepson." I hate that "step" label. I don't want him feeling as though I think of him any differently than I do toward my biological children. I want to minimize any insecurities, doubts, or fears Jordan might have regarding a sense of belonging, family, and foundation. I am proud to call him my son and delighted on the occasions he calls me "Dad."

Jordan is an adult now, but we get together with him whenever his schedule permits, mostly for birthdays and holidays, where we wind up celebrating at restaurants. When it's time to pay the bill and the server asks, "Separate checks?" My response is always, "He's with me."

Just as I am to the rest of our kids, I am an imperfect father to Jordan. Fortunately for Jordan, He has a perfect heavenly Father. So do you. So do I.

Five times in Romans 8, we too are called "children." We have been permanently adopted into God's family. We are heirs to the storehouse of spiritual riches afforded to His children. One of those riches is an antidote to fear:

> *"For you did not receive a spirit that makes you a slave again to fear, but you received the Spirit of sonship. And by him we cry, 'Abba, Father.'"—Romans 8:15 (NIV)*

In this verse, Paul is reminding us of the assurance we have in our "Abba Father," which translates as "daddy." Because of who God is, a tender-hearted, compassionate daddy caring for His children, we needn't worry about our salvation.

As our future lives are assured, so are our current lives. We no longer need to live in fear regarding our sinful nature. We know that the Spirit gives life (Romans 8:10). We know that the power the Spirit provides can put to death our old selves (verse 13). We also know that, as His children, we can live by that very same Spirit (verse 14). The lives God's children live now can be lived without fear.

Where our fitness is concerned, we should find great comfort in knowing that the Spirit is in us. As such, we are not slaves to our old selves. The "you" who botched it before does not have to botch it again. Your Father has emboldened you by His Spirit. You are no longer obligated to the compulsions you felt in the past. The failures you felt were your future destiny are powerless over you. You are not bound to obey the temptations that presently threaten you (Romans 8:12).

The Father of the family you have been adopted into gives you strength. He gives you a way out of these old mindsets, freeing you from fear and freeing you for victory. As His children, we not only give the glory to the Father, but also get to share in it (Romans 8:17).

The Spirit of Sonship has made us His children . . . His sons and His daughters. Our permanent adoption into His perfect family can alleviate our fears over our eternal heritage and our earthly living. Our adoption gives us a sense of belonging, of family, and of foundation. For our gracious, compassionate, loving Father is proud to call you His child, and is delighted when you call Him "Daddy."

Someday, we will appear before God the Father. When we do, rest assured that the Holy Spirit—the Seal and the Spirit of Sonship—will be there. He will mark us, vouch for us, and include us as His, saying, "They are with Me."

Prayer
Father, thank You for adopting me into your family. Will You please forgive me when I take for granted the power of your Spirit within me? Please help me live a life evident of my eternal heritage. Amen.

Meditation
I am in God's family.

Daily Spiritual Exercise
Practice "spiritual breathing" throughout the day. By now, it should start feeling a little more natural. You should also start feeling more equipped by having the practice of spiritual breathing in your arsenal. It is a wonderful means for relying on the Holy Spirit in your daily life. He is a gift your spiritual heritage entitles you to, empowering you on earth while you look forward to a perfect life in heaven.

"Finally, be strong in the Lord and in his mighty power. Put on the full armor of God, so that you can take your stand against the devil's schemes. For our struggle is not against flesh and blood, but against the rulers, against the authorities, against the powers of this dark world and against the spiritual forces of evil in the heavenly realms."—Ephesians 6:10–12 (NIV)

Citing Paul's command to "put on the full armor of God" regarding our fitness may seem like overkill. We're not deep in persecution in some country hostile to the gospel that is seeking to silence our faith permanently. We're talking about losing some weight, building some muscle, sleeping better, gaining energy, and feeling better. Right?

The moment we decide there are times we can take off the full armor of God, however, that's the moment we start losing. That's the very moment the devil's schemes are taking hold. The devil is cunning. He cannot win against God; therefore, he attacks God's people. He does this, in part, by trying to keep our mindsets focused on that which is seen. So we fixate on the scale or food or the gym as if they are the problem. Yet, if our struggle is not against flesh and blood, then a flesh-and-blood solution will never succeed against it.

The devil is constantly diverting our attention away from "the spiritual forces of evil." He wants to keep us in the wrong battlefield. He wants us focused on our flesh and blood. When we look at the struggle through a physical lens, we tend to react with physical efforts. Acting out of our strength with our measly defenses results in failure, every time.

Fortunately, we don't have to rely on ourselves. We are called to be readied and alert, and to "be strong in the Lord and in His mighty power." We are not told to stand strong out of our personal strength. The Lord, in all His wisdom and might, has fully equipped us.

This week, we'll look at various spiritual defenses and weapons we have at our disposal. As we do, we'll get some comforting reminders of what the Lord has done on our behalf. As with weeks before, we will see that it's about what He will do with our faith and obedience.

Remember, Satan cannot win against God. If we are strong in God's power, Satan cannot win against us either.

Daily Spiritual Exercise: Write Scriptures on sticky-notes.
Every day this week, you will be offered a passage of Scripture to equip you with your fitness. The verse might be a promise, an encouragement, a praise, or a prayer. Write it on a sticky note and put it somewhere you will see it often. Whenever you read it, pray that it would be true in your life. Scripture is one of our greatest weapons against the enemy. The more we are in harmony with the power of God's Word, the less susceptible we are to the enemy's attacks.

Remember, the struggle against flesh and blood is a distraction. The real battle is not against what is seen, but what is behind the scenes. So take comfort in the marching orders He has given us. Then fight confidently against the forces at work against us, for we have been given the blueprint for victory.

Week 6 Day 1 | *Full Armor of God: Flesh and Blood*

"For our struggle is not against flesh and blood, but against the rulers, against the authorities, against the powers of this dark world and against the spiritual forces of evil in the heavenly realms."—Ephesians 6:12 (NIV)

The struggle is not against flesh and blood? Well, when we are talking about fitness, it sure feels like flesh and blood. Getting daily exercise, eating healthy food, and fighting through the morning sleepies, definitely seems like a physical struggle. Certainly, in the most basic sense, it is. If we only examine the struggle on the surface, our fitness is nothing but flesh and blood. Leaving it there, however, is where we get in trouble. When we are oblivious to the bigger picture, Satan wins. He is working against you on a spiritual level by keeping your fitness focused only at a physical level.

Say you're having a rough day. Kids misbehaving. Stressful deadlines at work. Money tighter than usual. The house is a wreck, you have an argument with your spouse, and you get a flat. What's a typical reaction? Reach for some chocolate, right? Or a pizza? Blow off your workout. Flip channels, veg out, and stay up too late. Who wants to deal with tomorrow if it's anything like today?

All of those reactions are understandable. However, when we start to really dig into them, we can start to see the devil at work. What happens when we go to the pantry for comfort instead of our heavenly Father? We assign a role to food that it was not meant to fill. We also are resigning our Father from a role He is meant to fill. When we give in to lethargy, rather than exercising with the bodies He's given us, we trade healthy for lazy. We forgo a natural outlet for relieving stress in favor of an unproductive behavior that only compounds it.

Rather than seeking Living Water as our source of renewal, we might seek an escape in TV. That spring quickly runs dry, leaving us parched.

Or we are just not ready to face tomorrow. So we put off getting the sleep we need because the sooner we sleep, the sooner tomorrow comes.

When we do that, we're presuming on our efforts to handle it. Yet wouldn't life be more fulfilling if we experienced God being faithful to His promise that "his mercies begin afresh each morning?"

Do not misunderstand: food, TV, and relaxation, on their own, are not the issue. It's in going to them rather than our Father that we start seeing the "spiritual forces of evil" at work. More often than not, these habitual yearnings come not with a shove, but a nudge. A gentle prod to settle here. A whisper to give in there. A faint draw to something, anything, other than Jesus.

How then do we distinguish between benign desires and those that could have a malicious objective below the surface? First of all, we need to be aware of the devil's intentions. Merely being on guard will go a long way to protecting our hearts and minds. As 1 Peter 5:8 tells us, "Your enemy the devil prowls around like a roaring lion looking for someone to devour." However, when we're anticipating the attack, it's a whole lot harder for the devil to sneak up on us. That's Spiritual Warfare 101.

Secondly, know that the devil will use anything and everything he can to "steal and kill and destroy." If food will steal your attention from seeking God first, then the devil may distract you with a pint of Rocky Road. If TV will kill an opportunity to commune with your Father, the devil might remind you about an "important" basketball game "everyone" will be watching. Again, the devil's arsenal includes anything and everything.

Part of "anything and everything" includes taking gifts God has given us and distorting their intended use. Rather than enjoying something God meant for your pleasure, the devil tries to make you feel guilty about it. He will use good for bad, and bad for worse.

All of this would be quite discouraging if we weren't equipped to go on the spiritual offense. As we will see throughout this week, we have even more protection. We have far more weapons. We have incredibly effective tactics for waging a winning war against the forces of evil.

Always remember this: while the spiritual struggle is real, the battle is already won!

Prayer

Thank You that I am not alone in this struggle. Will You forgive me when I react like I am alone? Please help me be aware of the enemy and to rely on Your strength, which will fully equip me. Amen.

Meditation

Our struggle can be God's victory.

Daily Spiritual Exercise

1 Peter 5:8 says, "Your enemy the devil prowls around like a roaring lion looking for someone to devour." Put a sticky note of this verse on the object where this verse has the greatest application. Maybe the verse goes on the TV, computer, refrigerator, or mirror. It is up to you.

Then, whenever you read it, let it not just serve as a reminder of the spiritual forces against you in this world. Also remember that greater is the One who is in you than the one who is in the world (1 John 4:4). The spiritual struggles may start in the heart, but it's the same heart where God works and wins.

Week 6 Day 2 | *Full Armor of God: The Belt of Truth*

If I told you something just once, it may or may not hit home. If I said it again a few seconds later, though, you might start thinking it was important.

Now, if God says something once, hopefully He gets your attention the first time. However, in Ephesians 6:11 and in verse 13, we are told twice to "put on the full armor of God." There must be some significance to the repetition:

> *"Therefore put on the full armor of God, so that when the day of evil comes, you may be able to stand your ground, and after you have done everything, to stand. Stand firm then, with the belt of truth buckled around your waist . . ."—verses 13–14 (NIV)*

Notice also that Paul says to put on the "full" armor of God. We don't want to go into battle with only a shield or only a helmet. We want to be fully clothed and fully equipped, lest we give the enemy an easy point of attack.

The advantages of putting on the full armor of God don't stop there. Notice the order of events: "Therefore put on the full armor of God, so that when the day of evil comes . . ." Which comes first, the armor or the evil? The armor, of course. We want to be ready, so we put it on now. We don't wait for evil to come and then go grab our garb like Batman. We put our spiritual protection on and keep it on, a la Superman, because we expect evil to come. Verse 13 tells as much: "when the day of evil comes." It's not "if," it's "when." Since the evil will not stop until Jesus returns, we're given no indication to ever remove the armor.

Armor is composed of many pieces; the first one Paul mentions is the "belt of truth." Soldiers would wear belts, in part, to secure what would otherwise be a loose tunic. A loose tunic not only signified unpreparedness, it could also be a hindrance. Having baggy garments in the throes of battle make swift swings of the sword and shield that much harder. Of course, a belt also encircles the whole person.

What kind of truth is this belt? God's truth. Total truth. The truth of the Word of God. The truth in God's ability to do what God says He can do. The only truth that cannot be thwarted, compromised, or conquered.

Truth is rather underrated—more specifically, the ability to own a truth in your heart. We know in our heads that Jesus died on the cross for us. That makes us new creations. Our hearts, however, don't always live like this because we don't always feel like new creations. Or we don't act like this because we haven't fully accepted His grace. Or we don't behave like this because we don't allow Him to live through us. We don't allow him be the new creation in us . . . and for us. We just don't quite own the truth and implications of the cross.

Let me ask, if you botch your diet or skip out on a workout you know you needed, what happens? You feel like a failure and that you'll never get this fitness thing figured out. Then, heap on an extra helping of guilt for even feeling this way. If this is you, my guess is you've taken off the belt of truth, and the enemy has struck a blow!

Now the attack doesn't diminish the truth any more than clouds diminish the power, heat, and light of the sun. Victory is still His because truth says you're more than a conqueror. Truth says that you can do all things through Christ who strengthens you. Truth says there is no condemnation for those in Christ Jesus.

When you're continually clothed in that kind of life-giving truth, you start fully owning in. You start owning what God has done, is doing, and will continue to do. What the Lord continues, evil cannot overcome.

So wrap yourself in this truth: standing firm in God will always allow you to stand your ground.

Prayer

Father, thank You for enlisting me in the battle that You have already won. Will You forgive me when I take off the belt of truth? Please, in Your perfect way, allow me to both know and own the truth of who You are and what You have done for me. Amen.

Meditation

You are Truth.

Daily Spiritual Exercise

Take out a sticky note and write down this passage from Ephesians 6:13– 14a: "Therefore put on the full armor of God, so that when the day of evil comes, you may be able to stand your ground, and after you have done everything, to stand. Stand firm then, with the belt of truth buckled around your waist …"

Then place the sticky note somewhere that victory doesn't seem to find you. Oftentimes, this is the mirror.

Now every time you read the verse, pray that you could keep the belt of truth tied tightly around your waist. Pray also that you could own in your heart what that truth implies. For God is truth and by keeping Him in our heart and on our minds, we can win every battle.

Week 6 Day 3 | *Full Armor of God: Breastplate of Righteousness*

". . . with the breastplate of righteousness in place . . ."
—Ephesians 6:14b (NIV)

As part of the "full armor of God," Paul next instructs us to put on the "breastplate of righteousness."

Breastplates would have been made of leather, heavy linen, or a hammered piece of metal. They were designed to mold to the torso in order to protect the heart, intestines, and other major organs. While these are obviously important physically, it's what they represented in Jewish culture that's most interesting. The heart represented the mind, will, and disposition, while the intestines were the seat of emotions and/or feelings. Where does Satan most often attack? Our minds and our feelings. Paul wants us to be on guard against these attacks by donning a breastplate. Not just any breastplate: the Breastplate of Righteousness.

Righteousness is a tricky quality for Christians to understand. Rather than tackling the intent of the word, we tend to avoid it or abuse it. We often mistakenly default to "self-righteousness," which is never something God wants. Or we wrongly define it as the righteousness God has already ascribed to us by way of His Son becoming sin (2 Corinthians 5:21).

What Paul is referring to here is how we live out our righteousness in a practical sense. What role do we play to reflect the righteousness God assigned to us when His Son died for us? Our role is to live righteously by obeying His Word. To obey His word will require us to protect our hearts and minds, hence the need for the breastplate.

Where our fitness is concerned, this kind of protection begins by keeping our intentions pure. This takes us back to our goals for our fitness. Remember, for Christians, the goals of getting fit and the results of getting fit must not be synonymous. The results of getting fit are losing weight, getting stronger, having more energy, lowering blood pressure, having more confidence, and so on. These are perfectly fine things to achieve. When they happen, we can praise God for Him enabling us and we can enjoy the blessing of the benefit. However, we shouldn't work because of the benefit; we should work because of the benefactor . . . our Heavenly Father.

When our primary motivation, however, moves from "wanting to honor God" to "looking good in a bathing suit," things change. We've tainted our motives. When those kinds of thoughts creep in, we need to take them captive and make them obedient to Christ (2 Corinthians 10:5). This will likely require a daily surrendering of your mindset. You see, it's just like Satan to distract us by getting our fitness focused on the wrong things, such as results. If you look around, that's the way of the world . . . to look better. However, Romans 12:2 tells us, "Do not conform to the pattern of this world, but be transformed by the renewing of your mind." You need to protect your focus by protecting your mind. That starts by focusing on Christ and following His Father's word.

Protecting our emotions will also go a long way toward consistently honoring God with our bodies. Far too often feelings, not facts, determine our actions. We don't feel like working out, so we don't. We do this knowing we need exercise as a part of our plan to honor God with our bodies. Factually, we know we need to eat more produce and fewer processed foods. Yet, in moments of weakness, we feel like swinging by the drive-thru for a quick and greasy "value" meal. When a bad day hits, deep down inside we know for a fact we should seek comfort in Him alone. However, we feel like eating chocolate instead and so that's where we go, which only reinforces an unproductive spiritual life.

It doesn't have to be this way. Yes, God has established the very high benchmark for living, but He also supplied the power to live it out. We just have to be willing to fight. Like the soldiers of the day, we have to be always ready, armed, prepared, and protected. It's up to us to securely fasten the Breastplate of Righteousness in place. It's up to us to willingly rely on the strength He supplies. It's up to us to live according to the Word He gave us.

If we don't remain honest and upright, we can't honor God in our hearts. If we don't honor God in our hearts, we can't honor God with our bodies.

When we do remain upright, however, it's then up to the Lord's capable hands to see us through to completion. We can present it all back to the Lord and trust in Him to protect us. We can fully expect and rely on the promise found in Philippians 4:7: "And the peace of God, which transcends all understanding, will guard your hearts and your minds in Christ Jesus."

Prayer
Father, thank You for Your promise to provide my every need, including my protection. Will You forgive me when I leave my heart and mind unguarded? Please help me live a righteous life by living out Your word. Amen.

Meditation
Protect my heart. Protect my mind.

Daily Spiritual Exercise
Honoring God with our bodies begins by honoring God with our heart. The peace He provides will help keep our hearts protected. It will help keep our righteousness intact.

So write down Philippians 4:7 on a sticky note. Put the note somewhere you'll see it every day. In fact, you might make two of them and place one on each side of the door to your house. That way you'll see it when you leave and when you come home.

Let the verse be a reminder that He can and will help you with your fitness. More importantly, let it remind you that He can help you with your righteousness.

Week 6 Day 4 | *Full Armor of God: Feet Fitted With the Readiness of the Gospel of Peace*

When I first started doing any kind of committed running, I figured I'd buy a pair of trail shoes. That way I could run in the woods as well as on the street. If I were to buy road-running shoes, I wouldn't be able to take them on the trail. Or at least that was my thinking.

As I started putting in the mileage, however, my feet were not the least bit happy about the trail shoes. It wasn't just because my muscles weren't as strong as they needed to be. The design of the shoe provided the wrong kind of sole, the wrong kind of protection, and the wrong kind of fit. My body should have merely been adjusting to the running itself and taken slightly out of its comfort zone. The blisters and pain in my feet, on the other hand, shouldn't have been a part of the program.

Eventually, I got fed up enough to shop at a proper running shoe store. They took my measurements, filmed my gait and pronation, and I ran around the block in a few different pairs. I settled on what I thought were some ugly, overpriced sneakers . . . but it was love at first run. My feet felt so good, I would have paid twice the price.

My feet were able to function correctly, so my legs felt better too. In fact, my feet put my whole body in a better position to excel. While I never caught the running bug, when I do run, I run with the right shoe.

The appropriate shoe is important for an athlete, a job, or a favorite pastime. Proper footwear is even more important for soldiers. Their feet need to be fully equipped for the terrain on which they operate. They need to be protected from hostile environments. They must withstand heavy loads and, at times, great distances. Perhaps most importantly, their feet need to be ready to perform in an instant. A soldier's life can quite literally depend on both thinking and moving on their feet.

It's no wonder that Paul addresses the feet when he talks about putting on the full armor of God.

". . . and your feet fitted with the readiness that comes from the gospel of peace."—Ephesians 6:15 (NIV)

Paul is referring to the peace we have with God. If we have professed Christ as our Lord and Savior and asked for the forgiveness of our sins, we are at peace with the heavenly Father. Simply put, in Christ, we are at peace.

Consequently, if our feet are fitted "with the readiness that comes from the gospel of peace," not only do we have the assurance of God's love for us, but we also have His promise to fight battles for us that we can't win without Him.

That doesn't absolve us, however, from our responsibilities amid the fight. Our feet need to be ready to stand firm—dig in our heels and stay put, unwavering, and unafraid! We can be unafraid because God is the one taking care of business. We see this scattered throughout the Bible, where we are instructed to "stand firm" and watch God do the work. For example, Moses tells the Israelites this in Exodus 14:13: "Stand firm and you will see the deliverance the Lord will bring you today." God delivers when we stand firm.

We see this also in 2 Chronicles 20:17, before God defeats the Moabites and Ammonites on the king's behalf. King Jehoshaphat is told, ". . . stand firm and see the deliverance the Lord will give you, Judah and Jerusalem. Do not be afraid; do not be discouraged . . ." God defeats when we stand firm.

King David understood God's unassailability as seen in the famous Psalm 20:7, "Some trust in chariots and some in horses, but we trust in the name of the Lord our God. They are brought to their knees and fall, but we rise up and stand firm." God saves when we stand firm.

Jesus, of course, understood the importance of standing firm as He mentions it in three of the four Gospels, including Mark 13:13: "Everyone will hate you because of me, but the one who stands firm to the end will be saved." Again, God saves as we stand firm.

Paul makes his point again in 2 Corinthians 1:21–22: "Now it is God who makes both us and you stand firm in Christ. He anointed us, set his seal of ownership on us, and put his Spirit in our hearts as a deposit, guaranteeing what is to come." God helps us stand firm and guarantees when we do.

When our feet are fitted with the Readiness of the Gospel of Peace, He delivers. He defeats. He saves. He guarantees. In every fight you have with food. In every war you wage with a workout. In every battle against the bulge. If your feet are firmly planted in the peace that comes with God as your source of strength, hope, and faith, God does the rest and He gives the victory.

Prayer
Father, thank You for fighting my battles for me, and for winning them. Will You forgive me when I have weak knees, run away, or have misguided trust? Please help me to always remember that You are my source of victory. Amen.

Meditation
The armor of God helps me to stand firm.

Daily Spiritual Exercise
2 Corinthians 1:21 says, "Now it is God who makes both us and you stand firm in Christ . . ." This should be a great comfort. Yes, we are told to stand firm, but He even helps us with that.

Write down 2 Corinthians 1:21 on a sticky note and put the note where you will see it a lot. No, the battles we face aren't going to stop. Neither will the peace that comes with knowing the King will provide the victories.

Week 6 Day 5 | *Full Armor of God: Shield of Faith*

The word "faith" means different things to different people. For some, it's almost exclusively used in terms of self. "I know I can do it. I've got faith in myself!" For others, it has become this notion that everything will be handled with some kind of cosmic evenhandedness: "I'm not worried. I have faith it will all work out in the end."

For the Christian, there is no greater weapon, or form of protection, than our faith. Not our general, overarching faith or set of core beliefs, rather, our faith in Christ, specifically, is the source of our redemption and provision. That's why we shouldn't be surprised to read about a "shield of faith" instead of a shield of "joy" or "peace" or "righteousness":

> *"In all circumstances take up the shield of faith, with which you can extinguish all the flaming darts of the evil one."*—Ephesians 6:16 (ESB)

We can see the use of the word "shield" as symbolism throughout the Bible. God referred to himself as a "shield" in His covenant to Abram (Genesis 15:1). Moses referred to God as the shield of Israel in his final words to them (Deuteronomy 33:29). As seen many times in the Book of Psalms (perhaps most famously in Psalm 18:2), David was especially fond of referring to God as his shield . . . and for good reason. God had protected David from his enemies, most notably Goliath and Saul. Solomon also used such symbolism in Proverbs (2:7 and 30:5). As you can tell, it made good sense for God to be seen as a shield and a source of protection.

In early times, shields generally came in two sizes. There were small shields for hand-to-hand combat. There were full-body length wooden shields too. They would protect lines of soldiers from the barrage of arrows raining down on them as armies moved toward their enemy. These shields were soaked in water, so that when a flaming arrow came at them, the fire could be put out. We can quickly discern that Paul was referring to the full-body shields when he referred to extinguishing "flaming darts." A shield of that nature could both protect from the initial strike and prevent further damage from the arrows.

In order to stop an arrow, we first need to take up the shield. Like being fitted with the feet of readiness of the gospel of peace, we need to be prepared. When? Only part of the time, right? Just with some things? No! As verse 16 says, "In all circumstances." All the time, with everything, including your fitness . . . take up the shield.

So you can do what? Wait for the enemy to attack? Wrong! The enemy is already attacking. We take up the shield so we can take down the arrows. With it, we can disarm the evil one and his mission to derail our efforts to honor God with our bodies.

Which arrows? A few of them? The ones we get hit with most often? Only the ones we think are real problems? Absolutely not. They're all a problem and therefore we are told to extinguish "all" of them. This includes the lies you tell yourself: "I can't do that workout." "I'll cave again." "I'll never reach my goals." They are all flaming arrows and you can extinguish all of them.

Notice our role in the use of the shield of faith. God is not saying we are to be passive bystanders and wait for the shield to work magically. We play a part in our protection. We have to take up the shield in all circumstances and put out all the arrows being fired at us.

Therefore, our shield, our faith in Christ, should be both the backdrop and foreground of every decision, motivation, and inspiration. This faith requires a complete reliance, vulnerability, and expectation. The same faith also provides a God who has proven trustworthy countless times. Unending compassion. Unfailing love. Unparalleled power.

That's what makes this so interesting and so wonderful. Although taking up our shield of faith involves us, our faith doesn't rely on us. Our trust is in His trustworthiness. Our faith is in His faithfulness. As the writer of Psalm 91:4 says, ". . . his faithfulness will be your shield."

You see, the shield of faith protects and prevents. It deflects the burning arrows and it douses the fire before the damage starts.

The shield of faith both frustrates and fulfills. It hinders the evil one, but it honors the exalted One.

The shield of faith both demands you and delivers you. It requires you to use it, but it releases you from the results.

Take up your shield of faith. Keep it up, in all circumstances, against all arrows!

Prayer
Father, thank You for Your faithfulness. Will You forgive me when I fail to prepare, fail to act, or fail to rely on You? Please help me to always have my shield readied, but have my dependence on You. Amen.

Meditation
My shield of faith is strong because You are stronger.

Daily Spiritual Exercise
Find a place to put a sticky note with Psalm 91:4 on it, which reads, "He will cover you with his feathers, and under his wings you will find refuge; his faithfulness will be your shield and rampart."

As you pursue a healthier lifestyle, arrows will undoubtedly be fired your way. Be proactive. Take up your shield now. Then remember that your faith is in His faithfulness, and His faithfulness will protect you.

Week 6 Day 6 | *Full Armor of God: Helmet of Salvation*

The human brain is nothing short of astonishing. It consists of some 100 billion neurons, each with up to 10,000 synapses, and a network of 100,000 miles of blood vessels. The brain is a superhighway of information traveling insanely fast. It's the control center for the body's functions and movements, all of our intellectual activities, and our learning and memory. Powering our perception and behavior, our thinking and our emotions, the brain is the preeminent multi-tasker. In a classroom of other organs, it would be the standout overachiever.

Yet, as my parents taught me growing up, your biggest strength can be your biggest weakness. With all the potential for advancement, productivity, and good, we can also get caught up in the wrong things. We can battle mind games, under-examine, overthink, and be susceptible to both pride and defeat. That's why Paul would want our heads to be guarded, as well as our hearts:

"Take the helmet of salvation . . ."—Ephesians 6:17a (NIV)

Paul understood that Satan is a master gardener. He plants seeds of disbelief, discouragement, and pride that will have you questioning your salvation, your need for salvation, or both. These seeds are first sown in our minds. Then, they are watered, fed, and temperature-controlled that they might bear the rotting fruit of destruction. In order to keep the seeds from ever taking root, Paul highlights the need to keep your mind safe. That requires protection.

Fitness is certainly no stranger to mind games. It's easy to let our heads dictate our emotions. Before we know it, we're doing things based on how we feel. Even when that's not the case, there are other ways we intellectually sabotage our fitness.

Rooted in fear, discouragement is something most everyone faces during a fitness journey. The weight isn't coming off. The muscle isn't going on. The sleep is going down or the race times are going up. Whatever results you're hoping for, you aren't getting any closer to reaching them. Fear makes you doubt if it's worth it, if you're worth it, or if you'll ever get there: "Will things ever improve?"

The discouragement often leads to doubt—doubt as to whether you can maintain the workout schedule, eating plan, discipline, time requirement, and so forth. Or there's doubt as to whether the process will even work.

Perhaps thinking the science is wrong, you're doing it wrong, or your body is an anomaly. What begins innocently enough as merely questioning the process concludes with quitting.

Maybe it's the complete opposite: total pride. You've seen incredible progress. Now you think you can do more, faster, heavier . . . without accountability, without balance, and without the help of anyone. This can quickly backfire with injury, ego, regression, lost perspective, and lost relationships.

With each of these seeds Satan is planting, we need the protection our Father provides. If it's disappointment you are facing, pray that your helmet of salvation will be lined with the kind of encouragement only He can give. We know He can empower us with a sound mind (2 Timothy 1:7).

When you have doubts, pray that your helmet will provide the kind of assurance only God can give. We know that He can renew our thoughts and attitudes (Ephesians 4:23). When Satan attacks with the lies of self-reliance, pray that your helmet of salvation will be coated in humility. We must always recognize God is the one who equips us. Therefore, we would be wise to always keep Him involved at the center of our thought life:

> *"Keep falsehood and lies far from me; give me neither poverty nor riches, but give me only my daily bread. Otherwise, I may have too much and disown you and say, 'Who is the Lord?'"—Proverbs 30:8–9b (NIV)*

Discouragement, doubt, and pride all have something in common: missing or misplaced trust. Yet by filling our minds with Him, trust in Him naturally follows. When *we decide* to place our security in the Lord and the Lord alone, He provides protection. Proof is in Isaiah:

"You will keep in perfect peace those whose minds are steadfast, because they trust in you."—26:3 (NIV)

A mind at peace cannot be a mind drowning in discouragement, doubt, and pride. A mind full of Him cannot be full of anything else except Him.

Out of that peace we are reminded about how much He cares for us. How He provides for us. How He has saved us.

The helmet of salvation was offered with you in mind, so put it on. After all, if the Lord is that mindful of us (Psalm 8:4), how much more should we keep our minds full of Him?

Prayer

Father, thank You for the promise and gift of salvation in Your Son Jesus. Will You forgive me when I allow my mind to become a fertile field for the enemy? Please help me keep a protected and clean conscience, one focused on who You are and what You have done for me. Amen.

Meditation

My mind is Yours. I trust You to protect it with the helmet of salvation.

Daily Spiritual Exercise

Isaiah 26:3 says, "You will keep in perfect peace those whose minds are steadfast, because they trust in you." Write this verse on a sticky note and put it in a visible, high traffic area in your home.

Whenever you read it, pray that He would allow your mind to be steadfast on Him and the peace He gives. For when the truth of our salvation is foremost in our mind, we can rest in the security of His provision.

Week 6 Day 7 | *Full Armor of God: Sword of the Spirit*

The last piece of the coat of armor Paul instructs us to equip ourselves with is a sword. Not just any sword, a very special sword:

> "*. . . and the sword of the Spirit, which is the word of God.*"
> —*Ephesians 6:17b (NIV)*

The other pieces of the full armor we have discussed are used primarily for defensive measures. The Sword of the Spirit, however, is unique in its ability to function more than in just a defensive manner.

A skilled fighter uses his sword to do three things: defend, disarm, and attack. It would make sense then that only the inerrant Word of God would be that weapon for God's children. As we'll see, the sword of the Spirit has the ability to do the same three things.

Firstly, to prevent a sword from ever hitting them, fighters use their swords to block the incoming strikes. This requires fighters to have minds that are as quick as their hands. If they don't anticipate the direction, speed, or power of the coming blow, they won't move their hands in time to stop it. With a quick mind, however, expectant hands are readied for impact to prevent the opponent's sword from hitting its mark.

The Word of God acts as a perfect defense against the attacks of the enemy too. Proverbs 30:5 tells us that God's Word is a shield to those who seek refuge. When we are quick to use it, we will find that it's quick to protect us.

Secondly, a sword can be used to disarm the enemy. When two fighters are engaged in a swordfight, it's far easier to protect and attack when the opponent is weaponless. Knocking the sword out of an enemy's hands is part of the strategy. The stronger the fighter and the stronger the sword, the easier this is to accomplish against our foes.

There is no sword stronger than the Bible, no weapon more capable of disarming the enemy. We know this because Paul says in 2 Timothy:

"All Scripture is God-breathed and is useful for teaching, rebuking, correcting and training in righteousness, so that the servant of God may be thoroughly equipped for every good work."—3:16–17 (NIV)

As His servants training in righteousness, we can be "thoroughly equipped" and ready for every battle that comes our way. First John 2:14 reminds us that having and knowing the Word of God helps the fighter increase in strength: ". . . because you are strong, and the word of God lives in you, and you have overcome the evil one."

Lastly, we know that a sword can be used to attack. As an offensive weapon, it can put an end to a battle by putting an end to the enemy. Swords require precision, and an understanding of how, where, and when to thrust it into the vulnerable areas of an attacker. Certainly, the infallible Word of God can be used to end battles:

"For the word of God is alive and active. Sharper than any double-edged sword, it penetrates even to dividing soul and spirit, joints and marrow . . ."—Hebrews 4:12a (NIV)

Like the sword, the Word of God must be understood. We must learn how to apply it properly. Therefore, we pray for discernment and clarity, knowing also that the Word will nourish our spiritual growth (1 Peter 2:2). Then, we come into better and better understanding of the truth and power God has breathed into it.

Next week, we'll reach the halfway point of this fitness journey. You may have already noticed spiritual attacks increasing, as you aim to glorify Him more and more with your body. The enemy doesn't want God to have any glory of any kind.

To damper your progress (or discourage you because of your lack of it), a rising onslaught of jabs and barbs are coming at you. They're designed to knock you back, back you down, and bowl you over.

The good news is the enemy doesn't have the final say. He also doesn't want to see you reach for the Sword of the Spirit.

If we want to defend, disarm, and attack, we have to be warriors. We have to be quick, strong, and precise in our use of the Word of God. We do this recognizing, as David did, that the victory we will taste is not achieved by our efforts. It comes from the gracious love, compassion, and provision of our heavenly Father:

"I put no trust in my bow, my sword does not bring me victory; but you give us victory over our enemies, you put our adversaries to shame. In God we make our boast all day long, and we will praise your name forever."—Psalm 44:6–8 (NIV)

That's our battle cry! Grab your sword and stand firm. Praise Him and give thanks. No matter what happens this week in the fight for your fitness, He has given you the ultimate victory through His Son:

"But thanks be to God! He gives us the victory through our Lord Jesus Christ."—1 Corinthians 15:57 (NIV)

Prayer

Father, thank You for Your perfect Word. Will You please forgive me when I fail to cherish its beauty or apply its life-giving power to my walk with You? Please help me etch it onto the tablet of my heart, so that You will be glorified in my life. Amen.

Meditation

Your Word—the Sword of the Spirit—defends, disarms, and protects.

Daily Spiritual Exercise

Hebrews 4:12a says, "For the word of God is alive and active. Sharper than any double-edged sword, it penetrates even to dividing soul and spirit, joints and marrow . . ." Write that down on a sticky note. Then place the note on your nightstand, your steering wheel, computer monitor, or wherever you will see it often.

Remember that the versatility of the Word will win every time, but we must be ready to wield it.

WEEK 7 PREVIEW
Freedom

The greatest gift man has ever been given is free will. Without it, we would have no need for a Savior. We'd all be robots, preprogrammed to "love" God with insincere, systematic hearts. In light of free will, the love Jesus Christ displayed by dying on the cross for our sins becomes all the more remarkable. God gave us the ultimate freedom to accept or reject the ultimate act of love so that we could inherit the ultimate reward.

In His perfectly loving plan for us, God gave us minds of our own. He gave us freedom. This freedom goes unused by some believers. They don't truly understand it:

> *"But whoever looks intently into the perfect law that gives freedom, and continues in it—not forgetting what they have heard, but doing it—they will be blessed in what they do."—James 1:25 (NIV)*

Many believers have a hard time living free from the shackles of the flesh that the cross shattered. No longer must we be chained to our carnal cravings and the devastation that comes with them. A Christian's life is less restricted, not more. We can be freed from our old selves and the desires innate to sinful man. Desires that can never be satisfied for long. Desires that weigh us under, tear us down, and hold us back. Desires that suffocate freedom.

Yet even when living out the freedom the cross gives, sometimes those desires creep back in unnoticed. Before long, they've constricted some part of who we are. Some portion of our lives gets entangled in the chains of our sinful nature. The freedom we lived in is now less free.

This week we're going to get some reminders on what those freedoms mean for us, including for our fitness. As the week goes on, we'll see the perfection of the law that gives more and more freedom. We will begin to see how blessed we are because of it.

Daily Spiritual Exercise: Spend 3–5 minutes a day in adoration prayer.

Have you ever received a "Just Because" card—a note from someone who wanted to shower you with love for no other reason than because they think you're special? Aren't those awesome! I mean, special occasion cards are great, but because they're kind of expected, a little of the magic is lost. "Just Because" cards are given just because. The giver freely gives because they want you to feel cherished.

This week, practice adoring God . . . just because. Freely love Him. Freely praise Him. Freely acknowledge His greatness.

For three to five minutes a day, read a psalm. Sing a song. Pray a prayer. Ask for nothing. Tell Him He is everything. Spend the time doing nothing but adoring Him.

Week 7 Day 1 | *Freedom: From Guilt*

Gigi, our third child, is our butterfly. At six years old, she is a little on the shy side; she's happy on her own, playing in the imaginary worlds she creates. She has been blessed with a helpful heart, eager to give a hand any way she can. When she's not drying dishes, washing fruit, or cleaning up after her little brother, she's frequently fluttering from room to room—a touch here, a peek there, until finally she lands, settling on her own flower for a spell.

All that floating around, however, can get Gigi into some trouble. If she's not careful, she will find her way into things and places she shouldn't.

I can remember on more than one occasion finding Gigi uncharacteristically still. During such times, her wings are static, her demeanor stifled. When I ask her what's wrong, her usual warmth has been replaced by a cold reluctance. Behind her eyes, she's holding back pain.

I can sense her pain is self-inflicted. More often than not, I'll already know what's bothering her. On my better days, I'll gently wrap my arm around her small frame and pull her in close. I'll ask if she'd like to tell me what happened. Her eyes can no longer hold back the tears and with a little more prompting from me, she confesses to some form of disobedience.

We will then talk through what happened, why it happened, and a discipline is discussed. After she's taken ownership of her sin, asked for forgiveness, and we've prayed, her wings start flapping again. The guilt is gone and she's freely floating around the house once more.

Guilt can be productive. Gigi was convicted of her sin, which led to confession, repentance, and forgiveness.

Guilt can also be oppressive. It can change who we are and who He made us to be. Guilt turns Gigi from a butterfly into a knot on a log. Perhaps it turns you into an introspective mess. Or a slave to a "works" mentality. Or a fake. Or a . . .

Our Father has freed us from all guilt and the chaos it creates:

> *"Let us draw near to God with a sincere heart and with the full
> assurance that faith brings, having our hearts sprinkled to cleanse
> us from a guilty conscience and having our bodies washed with pure
> water."—Hebrews 10:22 (NIV)*

As Christians, we can draw near to God with a sincere heart. We can let Him wrap His perfectly loving arms around us and pull us in tight. He will remind us that our sins are forgiven and our minds purified of all guilt.

Unlike me, though, God doesn't have "better days." He only knows perfection. Out of that perfection, He washes our hearts clean. No more remorse about a food addiction. No more shame for making an idol out of exercise. No distress about not eating a perfect diet. No sorrow for past lethargy or indifference or poor body stewardship.

The sanctifying love of God does not stop there. He doesn't purify only part of our mind or wash only a portion of our heart. We are cleansed completely. Therefore, there's no guilt for any other area of our lives either.

So lean into Him. If you have something to confess, confess it. Then accept what comes next . . . the gift of guiltlessness. For when your heart and mind is on Christ, there's no place for guilt to reside.

Prayer
Father, thank You that You want me to seek You and that You will always listen. Will You forgive me for holding on to guilt that You have already freed me of? Please help me to always draw near to You. Amen.

Meditation
I draw near and You free me.

Daily Spiritual Exercise
Psalm 119:45 says, "I will walk about in freedom, for I have sought out your precepts." Perhaps reading Psalm 119 in its entirety can be a part of your adoration prayer for the day. As you pray, tell the Father how wonderful He is and how grateful you are for His love for you. Be sure to thank Him for the freedom He gave you in His son. For freedom in Christ is freedom from guilt. If sin is confessed, guilt has no home in the heart of a Christian.

Week 7 Day 2 | *Freedom: For*

Ever heard about the behavioral study where data was gathered on a playground? Surrounded by a fence, the playground was a flurry of activity for students in their free time. Swinging. Sliding. Laughing. Life was good.

Then, researchers removed the fence. When the kids went out for recess the next day, they stayed mostly huddled in the middle of the playground. Now unsure about exploring, they were apprehensive and uneasy.

The researchers put the fence back and the next day, all the running, playing, and carrying on returned. It was back to business as usual for the children. The fence gave them a sense of security. That security translated into greater confidence, and the fun followed.

At first glance, it would be hard to see how the fence boundaries gave the children freedom, but they did, and not just freedom "from" negative things, such as the temptation to wander off or the threat of dangerous people entering the playground. The boundaries also gave them freedom "for" things, such as exploring the playground, climbing on the equipment, and playing tag.

That's the flipside of freedom, and more specifically, freedom in Christ. Jesus doesn't only release us from the negative: bondage to sin, guilt, performance-based acceptance, the law of sin, etc. He liberates us for the enjoyment of the positive: love, joy, peace, patience, kindness, goodness, faithfulness, gentleness, and self-control, for starters:

> *"It is for freedom that Christ has set us free. Stand firm, then, and do not let yourselves be burdened again by a yoke of slavery."*
> *—Galatians 5:1 (NIV)*

This means that, as Christians, we can celebrate being released from the yoke of slavery. We can also take great delight in the blessings God has orchestrated for our pleasure.

Some people say that you should not merely try to eliminate a bad habit. If you do, you leave an empty spot for that habit to return. You'll be more likely to change your behavior if you replace the old habit with a new one.

Our mental outlook regarding our fitness should be no different. We are far too focused on what we are giving up: junk food, time, TV or Internet or books and magazines, money, energy, resources, etc.

Instead of focusing only on the sacrifice (i.e., junk food, time, TV, etc.), we should focus on the reward. We should replace the thoughts of what we're freeing ourselves from with thoughts of what we're freeing ourselves for.

We are freeing ourselves for things such as playing with our kids or grandkids without losing our breath. Savoring the countless all-natural foods God created for our taste buds to enjoy. Having sustained energy throughout the day. Minimizing potential injuries. Being less self-conscious in our swimsuit at the beach. Lessening the likelihood of being struck with certain diseases. Serving our neighbors, church, and community at a higher capacity. Running a mudder, 5K, or mini or full marathon. Or taking a well-deserved Sunday afternoon nap.

This kind of freedom—the freedom "for"—is part of His perfect plan for our lives, wherever we are. Second Corinthians 3:17 says, "Now the Lord is the Spirit, and where the Spirit of the Lord is, there is freedom."

Imagine! That same spirit resides in us, in our hearts. Wherever we are . . . freedom! The freedom He set us free for—the very freedom that lives in us—is a complete freedom . . . with two sides!

The "from" and the "for"—both are designed for our benefit. Both are designed for His glory.

Prayer

Father, thank You for not just freeing me from sin. Thank You also for freeing me to enjoy You, that You might be glorified. Will You forgive me when I fail to remember all that You've freed me to enjoy? Please help me to live a life characterized by the freedom You have given me. Amen.

Meditation

I am free for your glory.

Daily Spiritual Exercise

The Living Bible Translation of Psalm 34:4 says, "For I cried to him and he answered me! He freed me from all my fears." What great comfort that He answers and that He answers in favor of freedom.

Psalm 34 might be a good starting place for your three to five minutes of adoration prayer for today. It certainly is a great reminder of what the Lord is doing for us.

As you pray, remember that freedom in Christ is freedom to enjoy the life He has designed for us—a life lived with that design is the freest of all, and consequently where we will bring Him the most glory.

Week 7 Day 3 | *Freedom: From Performance*

I was recently on a national radio program discussing the relationship between faith, fitness, and finances. Shortly into the program, I was asked if I thought God was "displeased" with us if we're out of shape.

It's a good question. Whenever possible, I remind people that our fitness should be a response out of gratitude, not a sense of indebtedness. After all, it's not as if we could ever adequately pay Him back for all that He's done.

I responded with something along the lines of, "Let me be very clear: There's nothing we can do to add to God's love for us. It was already on display 2,000 years ago on a cross. Because of this, His love can't be added to nor can it be diminished. None of our efforts to get fit or be fit should be viewed in a way that we are trying to earn anything. We have to be careful to avoid a works mentality."

Avoiding a works mentality is vital for people to understand, so much so that we require an unusual task when visitors register on our website. Users are asked to print off the following "Letter From God" and post it somewhere they'll see it frequently:

> Dear Child,
> I love you just as you are.
> My love for you has already been established. My love for you has already been proven.
> My love for you has already been confirmed . . . determined . . . displayed.
> You can't add to my love, earn more of my love, or increase my love.
> **It is independent of you.**
> My love can't be diminished, tarnished, or lessened.
> **It is independent of you.**
> My love doesn't rely, depend, or hinge on you.
> **It is independent of you.**
> My love is unwavering, unfailing, and unending.
> **It is independent of you.**
> And because my love is perfect, I love you just as you are!
> — God

Today marks Day 45 in our fitness journey together. We're exactly halfway finished. That can be both exciting and disheartening.

Exciting because, hey, 45 days are under your belt. Disheartening because, whoa, after all this work, you're only halfway there . . . you have to do it for another 45 days!

This is the danger zone where people begin fizzling out of the journey. They're over the initial excitement. They've seen some results, but are potentially facing a plateau. By now, it's been established that living a permanently healthy lifestyle—while it gets easier—will always take work.

Planning ahead, squeezing in a workout, getting up earlier than you'd like, saying "no" to the wrong foods and saying "yes" to the right ones—it all takes time and effort. It all takes work. This work can grind on us spiritually, especially when we're operating out of our own effort, or out of the wrong mindset, like when we are exercising to avoid feeling guilty rather than to embrace feeling healthy.

That's why right now is one of the best times to reorient our thinking on why we're in this journey—why we're doing what we're doing. Remember, we should not be doing any of this on our own or to earn anything. Look at what Ephesians tells us:

> *"For it is by grace you have been saved, through faith—and this is not from yourselves, it is the gift of God—not by works, so that no one can boast."—2:8–9 (NIV)*

That should be music to your ears for a couple of reasons. For starters, we can't earn our salvation or all the love, care, and compassion that came with it. So, why wear yourself out trying to add to the gift that is already perfectly complete?

Also, when you operate out of a sense of indebtedness, you will merely be going through the motions with your fitness. You're going to feel bogged down and heavy, and burnout will most assuredly follow.

Yet, grace though faith saves us, not our works. Rather than us working out of our strength, we make room for God to work in us to bring glory back to Him. By approaching your fitness out of gratitude for the magnificent body He's given you, He can and will empower you.

Then, with the Lord as your motivation and power source for your fitness, you're not only free from performance, but you're also more free to enjoy Him in this process.

So, is God displeased with us when we are out of shape? I don't believe so. Is He, however, pleased with us when we, by His strength in us, honor Him with our bodies? I know so!

Prayer
Father, thank You for getting me this far. Will You forgive me when I try to earn your love rather than respond to it? Please remind me to keep You at the center of my fitness, my focus . . . my faith. Amen.

Meditation
I am free for you, that You might work in me and on me.

Daily Spiritual Exercise
Psalms 103–104 wonderfully portray some of the mighty works of the Lord. They might serve as a wonderful focus for your three to five minutes of adoration prayer. As you read them, let them be a reminder of all He has done with you in mind.

You can also remember all that Christ has done with you in mind, such as the freedom He has secured for you. Freedom in Christ is freedom from doing and freedom in living. Without the burden of trying to do it on our own, we can rely on Christ to do it for us . . . and we can enjoy Him more as He does.

Week 7 Day 4 | *Freedom: From Perfection*

Yesterday I shared about approaching our fitness from a place of gratitude rather than from a perspective of indebtedness. This frees us from the compulsion to perform. The lie of performance leads to the deception of perfection: it's a myth that you can and need to do something to add to or sustain the grace God offers.

Which reminds me: I have some good news and some bad news. First for the bad news: you'll never eat, exercise, or sleep perfectly. In other words, you'll never perfectly live out your fitness regimen. There are always ways to eat healthier, work out smarter, and sleep sounder. On one day, science will surely "discover the secret" that overnight fat loss comes through the consumption of some wonder-berry. The next day, a competing study will "discover the secret" that adding muscle comes through abstaining from that same wonder-berry.

Our bodies and the foods we are eating are changing constantly, as is the knowledge we have about both. So, living in a continuous state of flux makes living a perfect fitness life impossible.

Now for the good news: you'll never eat, exercise, or sleep perfectly. Why exactly is this good news? Because instead of obsessing about it, you can enjoy the process of getting fit by God's help. Rather than uselessly attempting to achieve fitness, you can marvel at the design He put into our incredible bodies. No more shouldering a burden so big that it prevents you from having any kind of satisfaction or fulfillment. You can celebrate the fitness victories He gives you.

Make no mistake: freedom from perfection does not free us from our obligation to honor God with our bodies (Romans 12:1; 1 Corinthians 6:19–20). It does, however, free us to enjoy the process of honoring God with our bodies without the fear of guilt and condemnation.

Perfection, on the other hand, is an illusion. It stems from and leads to pride, which, at its heart, is the inability or unwillingness to fully embrace His grace. You see, grace doesn't only require the acceptance of His unmerited favor, but it also requires the admittance of our unmitigated need. We certainly need Him as our Savior and the grace He offers for the forgiveness of our sins that we might inherit eternal life. Yet that's just the beginning, as our need doesn't stop there.

He came to give us life and have it to the full (John 10:10). In order to experience "to the full," we need to rely on Him beyond redemption. We need to rely on Him for daily regeneration, to empower us throughout our lives, not just save us at the end of them. When we're unable or unwilling to recognize our need for Him to be the perfect source of our efforts, futility ensues. We'll resort to working out of the imperfection of our own efforts.

I have some more good news. Once you fully accept God's grace, not only is He honored in it, He will empower you through it. Why? To bring glory to Christ. This is something Paul understood quite well. The Lord allowed Paul to be tormented, but when Paul asked for relief, the Lord responded:

> *"Each time he said, 'My grace is all you need. My power works best in weakness.' So now I am glad to boast about my weaknesses, so that the power of Christ can work through me."—2 Corinthians 12:9 (NLT)*

All Paul needed was God's grace. That's all I need. That's all you need. As Paul goes on to say in verse 10, we know that God makes us strong in our weakness. That's the power of Christ working in us!

Again, our strength—God's grace—requires us to recognize our weakness. That's why James reminds us that God gives His grace generously, but He gives it to the humble (James 4:6).

In God's ultimate sovereignty, He offers a relational love that is able to empathize with us in our weaknesses:

> *"This High Priest of ours understands our weaknesses, for he faced all of the same testings we do, yet he did not sin. So let us come boldly to the throne of our gracious God. There we will receive his mercy, and we will find grace to help us when we need it most." —Hebrews 4:15–16 (NLT)*

We are not alone. The One who equips us in our weaknesses is able to do so, in part, because He understands our weaknesses. Jesus was one of us, knows the trials we experience, and the temptations we face. This includes the temptation to try and live perfectly apart from the Father. However, we can go to Him and go boldly. There we can expect to find a gracious God who gives generously out of His love according to our need.

It's ironic that the stronger we are on our own and the harder we try, the worse off we are. It's not surprising to Satan, though, which is why he encourages this destructive loop. The more independent we become, the less we believe we need God. The less we believe we need God, the greater our pride.

The cycle continues. The greater our pride, the greater our independence becomes, as does the pressure we feel to perform. After all, we should be able to handle it, right? Then, the greater the pressure to perform, the greater our obsession for getting it exactly right . . . for perfection; which, remember, cannot be attained by human efforts.

Only through the death of Christ on the cross can we be made perfect in the eyes of the Father (Colossians 1:22). Then, someday, when we're united with Him, He'll give us new, perfect bodies of our own (2 Corinthians 5:1–5).

Until then, any perfection that exists in us is a reflection of Christ through us.

Living in Christ gives us the freedom to rely on the only perfect thing. Out of that perfection, His perfection, we have grace to make mistakes but the power not to:

> *"Sin is no longer your master, for you no longer live under the requirements of the law. Instead, you live under the freedom of God's grace."—Romans 6:14 (NLT)*

A grace that is freely given. A grace that is never earned. A grace that is perfect. A grace that gives life. A grace that gives freedom.

Prayer

Father, thank You for the grace of the cross. Will You forgive me when I seek any kind of perfection apart from You? Please help me to rely on the grace You give. Be the strength in my weakness and allow me to enjoy the process of honoring You with my body. Amen.

Meditation

Where His grace abounds, freedom reigns.

Daily Spiritual Exercise

Psalm 19:7 says, "The law of the Lord is perfect, refreshing the soul." When we realize how perfect only the Lord is, that there's no pressure on us to be perfect, it too is refreshing. The weight is off. The burden is light.

Perhaps Psalm 19 is a good starting off point for your three to five minutes of adoration prayer. As you pray and praise Him, remember His ways are true. His laws are right. His grace is sufficient and His power is perfected in our weakness.

Week 7 Day 5 | *Freedom: From Bondage*

We live in a residential neighborhood, but it's off the beaten path a little, surrounded by cornfields and some farmland. Our house is at the end of a cul-de-sac. It backs up to a family farm with some acreage for horses and chickens. One of the many perks to my job as a writer and fitness coach is I get to work from home. I have an office, but, if it's nice outside, I really enjoy working from our screened-in porch. It overlooks our backyard and our neighbor's fields and feels a little like being in the country.

Screened-in porches are great, but they're not impenetrable for insects; at least ours isn't. Whether through the floor of the decking or the ever-widening crack by the door, bugs find their way in somehow. Not small bugs either. Unless it's a wasp, I don't mind too much. In fact, I welcome the company, especially the bumblebees. They're too loud to sneak up on you. They're friendly enough to pet. They're great for the flowers. They just seem to have more personality than most bugs.

The problem for our bumblebees is that they trap themselves. They find their way into our porch, but have no clue how to get out. So, they end up crawling around the mesh screen trying to find an exit. When they have no luck with one screen, they may try another (or at least they think they're trying another). Too bad—they're stuck. They're inside looking out, sensing freedom without being able to experience it.

Fortunately for the bees, I've mastered the art of restoring their freedom. I take a plastic cup, turn it upside down, and place it just above the bee, coaxing them inside. Once they are in, I open the door to the backyard, give the cup a little shake and out fly the bees. Ahhhh, the sweet taste of freedom.

Yet there are still two issues for my little friends. First, when I'm trying to help them, they're not super happy about it. They get mad and buzz at me. They flap their wings a million miles a minute and try to crawl around the cup or fly out of it altogether. Eventually, I convince them that my way is better than theirs and they're released into the wild. It just doesn't happen without resistance.

The other issue is my bumblebee friends always seem to come back. Sure, some of them are first-timers, but I know a bunch of them are repeat offenders. They incarcerate themselves repeatedly. If I don't free them, they'll never touch another flower again.

We can be that way. We can be bumblebees. In fact, the Apostle Paul had to deal with a lot of bumblebees in his ministry.

These bees wanted to confine themselves to being justified by the works of the law that lead to sin and death. They needed to be told that justification through faith leads to freedom and life. That's exactly what we see Paul tell the church of Galatia: that freedom is found in Christ and Christ alone. We have dealt with this, but it's worth repeating:

> *"For freedom did Christ set us free: stand fast therefore, and be not entangled again in a yoke of bondage."—Galatians 5:1 (ASV)*

The thing that is so seductive about the law of sin is that it's familiar. We're born with that sinful nature, after all, so it's no mystery as to why we are drawn to it. Our sin is not new to us and therefore, we find it very comfortable. We revert to it time and time again because we know it so well.

Notice what Paul says. First, he tells them to "stand fast." Be strong, resolute, unwavering. No matter how tempting . . . stand fast.

Then he says to them, "be not entangled again in a yoke of slavery." He doesn't say, "if you can avoid it" or "give it a shot." In other words, it's a choice. It doesn't have to happen; we have a say in the matter. Like the bumblebees, we can roam free. We can have victory.

There can be bondage where your physical and spiritual health are concerned. Whether food or lethargy or whatever temptation is drawing you to the porch, it's holding you back. Doing what you want may seem like freedom but, like the bee on the screen, you're not truly experiencing it. You're inside looking out.

Unlike our friend the bee, we have a choice. We know the way out. We have Christ, who broke the yoke of bondage. We have the Holy Spirit, who gives us victory in our fitness struggles. We just need to submit and let Him work in us.

Now there will be times when you do find yourself back on the porch. Fortunately, God is there to rescue us. Don't buzz, flap, and try to fly away when He is trying to help. His way is better. His way is life. His way is freedom.

Ultimately, His way will enable you to stand fast, stay out of the porch, and fly free. Bzzzzzzzzzz!

Prayer
Father, thank You for helping me off the porch. Will You forgive me when I'm drawn to the things that hold me back from truly experiencing You? Please give me eyes for You, the only true freedom. Amen.

Meditation
Because of You, I will stand fast. By You, I will not be entangled.

Daily Spiritual Exercise
Psalm 18 speaks of the Lord's deliverance of David. There are some wonderful descriptions David uses to describe the Lord's work in His life. The beauty of it is, the Lord does these same things for us today, including freeing us from that which entangles. Read Psalm 18 as a part of your three to five minutes of adoration prayer.

As you do, give thanks for His son. Living in Christ gives us freedom from our old ways, the ways that held us back. That held us down. That held us captive.

No longer. Thanks to Jesus who freely gave His life, we may now freely live.

Week 7 Day 6 | *Freedom: From the Law of Sin*

I'm writing this on the Fourth of July, when our great country celebrates the adoption of the Declaration of Independence in 1776. Independence Day is the perfect name for it. We had declared our independence from Great Britain and established sovereignty as our own nation. We got our own form of government, laws, and rights. Now, we take this day every year to observe the meaning of this historic day.

We also use the Fourth of July as an opportunity to honor the military who sacrificed to preserve our freedoms. Hopefully, we stop to recognize God's role in it all. As John Adams wrote to his wife two days before Congress approved the declaration, "It ought to be commemorated as the day of deliverance, by solemn acts of devotion to God Almighty." Here we are nearly 250 years later still celebrating. We gather for picnics and parties, food and games, family reunions and fireworks in a national recognition of our heritage.

Well before our independence was secured, it was a far different story. The ideals that prompted the formation of a new nation were under the subjection of a hostile leadership, one that discouraged the various liberties we now hold dear. The dreams and aspirations of many could not be fulfilled while under the oppression of that form of government. Not under the rule of that kind of law.

Some brave men and women who could no longer stand the status quo of helplessness and condemnation sought change. They needed freedom from the law of their day.

We, too, need freedom from the law, but not the law from which our founders fled. If we want freedom, true freedom, we need release from the law of sin and death. Christ provided that unique freedom by His work on the cross. Before Christ came, we were bound to the law and slaves to our sin. Then, by His death and resurrection, we ourselves have "died to the law" through the body of Christ and risen from our dead bodies of sin. Jesus changed everything. He broke the chains that shackled us and in their place, He gave us true freedom:

*"But now, by dying to what once bound us, we have been released
from the law so that we serve in the new way of the Spirit, and
not in the old way of the written code."—Romans 8:6 (NIV)*

With that freedom in Christ comes freedom from the old way of things: freedom from the flesh (Galatians 5:13), freedom from accusation (Colossians 1:22), freedom from sin (Romans 6:6–7), and freedom from the yoke of slavery (Galatians 5:1).

We have been delivered from death. No longer sentenced to be slaves to our old sin nature, we are now to live as God's slaves (Romans 6:22).

That's the interesting thing about this. The independence we have in Christ requires total dependence *on* Christ. We live by Him, for Him.

When we do that, we are freed from condemnation and are given life:

*"Therefore, there is now no condemnation for those who are in
Christ Jesus, because through Christ Jesus the law of the Spirit
who gives life has set you free from the law of sin and death."
—Romans 8:1–2 (NIV)*

Your body was designed to move and God intended for you to have fun moving. Your mouth was designed to taste and God intended for you to enjoy eating. Your body was designed to rest and God intended for you to enjoy sleeping. From the beginning, He gave us the ultimate freedom to enjoy our lives and all the gifts He gave us. Those gifts, however, can take precedence over the Giver and very quickly we can become slaves to the law of sin.

God, nevertheless, gave us more gifts because of His gracious love for us. His first gift, Jesus, freed us from death. The second gift, the Holy Spirit, freed us to live abundantly. No longer slaves to the law, we are slaves to the Spirit, where freedom lives:

*"Now the Lord is the Spirit, and where the Spirit of the Lord is,
there is freedom."—2 Corinthians 3:17 (NIV)*

As great as the impact of Independence Day, dependence on Christ is greater still. The freedom represented by the Fourth of July pales in comparison with the freedom we have in Christ.

Prayer

Father, thank You for allowing me to live in this great country. Thank You even more for the freedom I get when I live for You. Will You forgive me when I allow myself to be enslaved by my flesh? Please help me to never abuse that freedom but rather always depend on You as my source of strength and hope. Amen.

Meditation

I live for You, by You.

Daily Spiritual Exercise

Romans 8:1–16 provides a unique opportunity to adore the Father, Son, and Holy Spirit.

Read each verse, one at a time. After each verse, pause to reflect on the implications it has for your life. Then, praise Him for the blessings those verses offer.

For instance, Romans 8:1 says, "Therefore, there is now no condemnation for those who are in Christ Jesus," So perhaps your adoration prayer goes something like: "Wow, Father! You are so good to me to share Your son Jesus with me. Now, I get to be in Him and Him in me. As if that's not enough, You no longer condemn me because of Jesus in me. No sin. No flaw. No failure. Nothing of mine is condemned by You any longer because of Jesus. Thank you. I am undeserving but am eternally grateful."

As you go about your three to five minutes of adoration prayer, let it be a comfort knowing you are free. You are no longer bound by the law that leads to death. You are free. Dependence on Christ has led to the ultimate freedom. You are free!

Week 7 Day 7 | *Freedom: From Our Old Identity*

Have you ever run into people after having not seen them in years? Perhaps you haven't seen them since high school or even childhood. You start talking and before long, you have one of two revelations.

The first is that they are exactly how you remember them. They have the same loud laugh, they're still a die hard sports fan, and they're still striving for the same empty pursuits. You're amazed at how, after all these years, they haven't changed a bit.

Or they are nothing like what you remember. The snotty cheerleader with a wild reputation authors a popular teen blog, teaching the values of purity and self-respect. Or the former bully is now a loving, stay-at-home dad of five who volunteers weekends with Habitat for Humanity. This time, you're amazed because after all those years, they aren't a bit the same.

Saul would fall into this second category. If you ran into him after his "road to Damascus" experience, you would have been in utter shock. The man you remembered was previously known for his mission to destroy the church. He approved of stoning Christians. He dragged men and women from their homes to throw them in jail. He threatened the lives of disciples, increasing persecution to the greatest degree. That's the Saul you remember, but he doesn't even go by that name anymore. It's Paul now.

Paul was now the prolific writer of roughly half of the 27 books of the New Testament. A captivating preacher, converting the lost, and building the church he formerly sought to tear down. A generous traveler, risking life and limb to spread the message of the love of Jesus. Possibly the most influential Christ-follower in the New Testament and arguably the most humble. Now after all these years . . . Paul wasn't a bit the same.

When we become Christ-followers, we are freed from who we were. We surrender our old lives and get new identities in exchange. Saul became Paul. Thus, Paul no longer lived in such a way that his old identity determined his new life.

Once Saul was converted, he didn't slip up and start persecuting

Christians again. He didn't stop and say, "Well, because I've always been a persecutor, I guess I always will be." He was freed from that old identity and it was no longer his struggle.

Too often, we let our past become our identity. We let our struggles define us. When they define us, they control us. This constantly happens with our fitness: "I've quit every program I've started . . . what's one more?" "I guess I'll just be overweight all my life." "It's not like I'm on drugs . . . at least my fitness addiction is good for me." Because it's who we've been, we let our struggles decide who we'll continue to be.

Paul would have a lot to say about that. If there's one thing he persecuted after his conversion, it was the old identity. Three times in the New Testament, he does just that. He reminds us that our old self, our old identity, has no business in the life of a Christ-follower. We see it in Romans 6:6, as he colorfully portrays what happens to our former identity, saying, "For we know that our old self was crucified with him so that the body ruled by sin might be done away with, that we should no longer be slaves to sin."

In Colossians 3:9–10, Paul portrays the old and new selves as if they're garments: "Do not lie to each other, since you have taken off your old self with its practices and have put on the new self, which is being renewed in knowledge in the image of its Creator." Because of who God says you now are, you are freed from having to wear your old, sinful self any longer.

Then in Ephesians we see that, because of who God is in us, we are becoming like Him:

> *"You were taught, with regard to your former way of life, to put off your old self, which is being corrupted by its deceitful desires; to be made new in the attitude of your minds; and to put on the new self, created to be like God in true righteousness and holiness."—4:22–24 (NIV)*

Did you notice what preceded the "new self"? That we are made new in the "attitude of our minds." God didn't just repair an old broken mind. Our mindset, our thoughts, and our attitudes are new, fresh out of the box!

While it's hard to comprehend, understand this: our math is not God's math. We are not the sum of our past, present, and future. We don't deserve our future. Our ways are not His ways. Where we find defeat, He finds victory. Where we see waste, He sees purpose. Where we see the same old, God gives us the brand-new.

Don't resign yourself to your struggle! Who you were is not who you are. It's certainly not who you have to continue to be. God is in the freedom-giving business and He has freed you now and for all eternity.

Prayer
Father, thank You for not seeing me the way I oftentimes see myself. Will You forgive me when I let my struggles define me rather than Your love? Please continue to renew the attitude of my mind. Help me live out the new self, created to be like You. Amen.

Meditation
My mind is new because of You.

Daily Spiritual Exercise
Psalm 136 is a wonderful chapter, perfect for your three to five minutes of adoration prayer. I want you to do something a little different as you go through it.

Each of the 26 verses ends with "His love endures forever." After you've read each verse, add to your prayer, "He has freed me from _____," filling in the blank with an attribute of your old self.

Then I want you to pause and give thanks for that miracle, reflecting on the amazing work God has done in your life.

Through this process, you will be reminded that because of who He is, who you were is not who you are. Therefore, you no longer live like you once did. You now live truly free.

Promises in the Bible

Ever made a promise to someone and then broken it? "I'll take out the garbage when I get home." "I'll play with you when I'm done on the computer." Perhaps worst of all, "I'm so sorry to hear that . . . I'll pray for you." We mean well, but don't deliver.

Ever made a promise to God and broken it? "I'll start being more consistent in my quiet times." "I'll give You more of my income." We sing in church, "I surrender all," but deep down inside we hold onto things. Or we'll belt out a heartfelt, "Where you go, I'll go. Where you stay, I'll stay. When you move, I'll move. I will follow." Yet we go someplace else, stay somewhere else, and chase something else. We mean well, but don't deliver.

The Bible is packed with promises from God to us. Unlike us, however, He doesn't break His promises:

> *"God is not human, that he should lie, not a human being, that he should change his mind. Does he speak and then not act? Does he promise and not fulfill?"—Numbers 23:19 (NIV)*

That means when God says He will direct our path, He will. When He says He heals the broken-hearted, He does. When He says that He is the same yesterday and today and tomorrow, He is.

What great comfort! The assurance of His promises equips us to tackle the issues in our lives with confidence. Whether our troubles are resolved or not, He will be there . . . unchanged. Be it fitness or financial, relational or occupational, emotional or spiritual, clinging to the truth of His promises sustains us.

In other words, He doesn't just mean well . . . He delivers.

Daily Spiritual Exercise: Meditate on God's promises.

For five minutes each day, you will be given a promise of God to meditate on, along with a corresponding verse. During this time, no music, other reading, distraction . . . or any of that. Merely meditate in silence for five minutes.

See what the Lord impresses on your heart.

Week 8 Day 1 | *Promises in the Bible: Mercies*

Last night was a night like any other. We plowed through the normal homework-dinner-hangout-bedtime ritual common to most families. The kids were fast asleep. My wife and I chatted about the day's events. It was late and before I knew it, she was asleep too. I read for a bit, then went to bed, thinking back on my day, and making plans for tomorrow.

I woke up to a day unlike any other. We had been hit with a snowstorm. The trees appeared as if they had been dipped in white chocolate. The neighbor's old rickety fence was now trimmed in white, somehow looking quaint. The snow was not so much falling down as it was racing sideways in blurry bits. At times, the wind would pick the snow up off the ground and throw it several yards away, rearranging the landscape repeatedly . . . as if the wind were sculpting, not merely blowing.

Then, every so often, the snow slowed. From chaos to calm, the mood instantly went from a minor chord to a major. Visibility restored briefly before the fury returned. There was still beauty in the chaos, just a beauty of a different kind.

What was unique about the morning wasn't that it had snowed, because it was snowing a lot this winter. It wasn't how it snowed, in fits and starts—nothing all that uncommon about that either.

What was unique was that the snowstorm wasn't on my radar. I had no idea we were due for any snow of any kind. I certainly didn't anticipate school closings, gymnastics classes being cancelled, and poor road conditions.

The morning reminded me of probably the most famous verse in Lamentations:

> *"The faithful love of the Lord never ends! His mercies never cease.*
> *Great is his faithfulness; his mercies begin afresh each morning."*
> *—3:22–23 (NLT)*

As the NIV puts it, ". . . for his compassions never fail. They are new every morning."

There's a difference between the morning's snow and this verse. The difference is that God should be on our radar. Every day, His compassions should be expected. What comfort! Every morning, He covers our sins. Every day, He wipes our sin clean. For all time, He has made us as pure as it was outside that morning: "Though your sins are like scarlet, they shall be as white as snow" (Isaiah 1:18).

The snowstorm also reminded me of when I was in school. Whenever I made mistakes, which was a lot, I'd flip the pencil around to correct them. A frenzied rub of the eraser and the lead came up, leaving behind a trail of eraser crumbs. A quick brush of the hand, a hefty blow on the paper, and specks of eraser scattered like a fast-falling snow. My paper became new again.

That is our God! That is His promise to us. We make plans, as I did the night before the snow. He then takes our plans and makes something beautiful out of them. He takes the chaos that is our fast-moving lives and makes something scenic from them. He takes the sin in our lives, erases it by the blood of Christ, and makes us new again.

God does this every . . . single . . . day. Furthermore, if He can do this with our sins, should our health present any real issue for him? When we botch our diet, we can start fresh the next morning. When we miss our workouts, we can start with a clean slate the next day. When we deprive our bodies of sleep tonight, He can give us the discipline to go to bed earlier tomorrow.

Put it on your radar. Revel in it. His mercies are . . . new . . . every . . . morning. Making us white as snow. Giving our old feeble fence character. Bringing our dormant trees to life. Covering the landscape of our lives and sculpting it into a beauty of a different kind. The kind in which God is glorified.

Prayer

Father, thank You, thank You, thank You for the daily renewal in our lives that You provide. Will You forgive me when I fail to remember Your mercy and compassion? Please help me to be merciful to others, as You have been so very merciful to me. Amen.

Meditation

Your mercies are new every morning.

Daily Spiritual Exercise

Today, you are going to meditate for three to five minutes on Lamentations 3:22–23. As you do, think about each word and the implications it has for both your fitness and your life in general. For instance, this passage uses words like "faithful," "love," "never ends," "mercies," and "afresh," all in reference to our Father. Consider the glorious consequences these words mean for you.

As you think through this great news, you'll be reminded that His mercy doesn't stop at covering our mistakes. His mercy gives us power to not make any more of them. Every day, day after day, this can reshape our lives . . . like snow on a landscape.

Week 8 Day 2 | *Promises in the Bible: Prayer*

Ever pray and then wonder if it were going to do any good? Ever knelt down and bowed your head, but felt disconnected, as if your prayers were just drifting off into the ether? Ever had prayers go without an answer of any kind?

This is an interesting dynamic, really. Most of the time, we have no trouble accepting that the Bible is true—that it's God-breathed, that it's the Word of Life. Then we turn around and question what the Bible says about prayer. We might not see it that way, yet that's what happens when we doubt the strength or usefulness of our prayer life.

The Book of James should encourage you as it proves the power of prayer:

> *"The prayer of a righteous person is powerful and effective."*
> *—5:16b (NIV)*

"Effective" is translated from the Greek word *energeō*, from which our English word "energy" is derived. I love that! *The Message* paraphrases it like this: "The prayer of a person living right with God is something powerful to be reckoned with."

God's Word to us promises that there is authority in our prayers. They get things moving. They get results. Our prayer is the fuse and He is the dynamite.

Still not convinced? Consider where this portion of the verse appears. It's sandwiched between a calling to be spiritually healed—". . . pray for each other so that you can live together whole and healed"—and the reminder of Elijah's prayer for an act in the physical realm: ". . . Elijah, for instance, human just like us, prayed hard that it wouldn't rain, and it didn't . . ."

Physical. Emotional. Spiritual. There is nothing off-limits for the power of prayer.

Make no mistake. Our prayers are powerful not because of anything we do or who we are. Remember, we're just the fuse. It's because of who He is and what He can do. Therefore, we can approach Him with an honest, upright, and believing heart. Then God is eager to respond, doing what only He can.

That's why James also reminds us to quit questioning what prayer can do:

> *"But when you ask, you must believe and not doubt, because the one who doubts is like a wave of the sea, blown and tossed by the wind. That person should not expect to receive anything from the Lord. Such a person is double-minded and unstable in all they do."—1:6–8 (NIV)*

No mincing words there. We need to drop the doubting of what we're doing when we kneel before the God of all creation. Quit questioning the effectiveness of presenting our requests to Him. Earnestly seek His will for your life, His wisdom for your mind, and His love to fill your heart. He delights in answering you. He is all about His glory. You can fully trust Him with your prayers, as you also trust the truth of His character, purposes, and promises.

Fitness is a struggle for so many people. Whether it's finding the time, desire, energy, discipline, balance, whatever the case, fitness can be a stumbling block. Our response may be to pray for help, but in our heart of hearts, we don't expect it to come. We don't expect an answer. We don't believe there is dynamite on the other end of the fuse.

Worse yet, we dump water on the fuse after it has been lit. We don't really want an answer to our prayer because it might mean giving up _____. Or we fail to listen for an answer. We don't consider the words of a loved one or examine Scripture with a truly open mind. Instead, we go about our days, too busy or unwilling to listen. Or maybe we ignore the answer we are given. We push aside that little nudge in our hearts and fail to follow through in obedience. We are double-minded. Unstable.

Before we know it, we are letting our struggle define us. That's why our prayers need to be offered with a clean heart—with pure motives, earnestly. God knows us better than we know ourselves and He can discern our intent. Yet, out of our vulnerability, we can approach Him void of pretention, full of confidence.

Prayer is one of our greatest tools for good and most effective weapons against the enemy. We should wield it with great confidence.

It knows no limits. Prayer is bound by nothing. God has the power to change anything and we have the privilege to approach Him about everything. We would be wise to do so, and to do so with confidence.

Prayer

Father, thank You for giving us access to You through prayer and for the delight You take in listening. Will You forgive me when I go through the motions with my prayer life? Give me a pure heart, Father, to believe and not doubt. Lord, I want to trust not only that You hear me but that You'll help me. I want to trust in your greater purposes for the countless things I do not know, see, or understand. Amen.

Meditation

My prayers are effective and powerful because God hears and answers.

Daily Spiritual Exercise

Today you are going to meditate for three to five minutes on Philippians 4:6–7, which says, "Do not be anxious about anything, but in every situation, by prayer and petition, with thanksgiving, present your requests to God. And the peace of God, which transcends all understanding, will guard your hearts and your minds in Christ Jesus." As you meditate on these promises, pray for the faith to believe them.

Remember that when we pray, God is listening and He is more than able to help. Then, when He does, we have to be ready to act on His provision.

Week 8 Day 3 | *Promises in the Bible: Help in Our Weakness*

In the introduction of the book, I said the following in regard to this 13-week fitness journey: ". . . this is first a spiritual issue and that honoring God with our bodies begins by honoring God with our hearts." It's for this reason we frequently talk about the heart and what our reliance on the Holy Spirit, our heart pilot, should look like.

Yesterday, we talked about the power of praying confidently and with a clean heart. Tomorrow, we'll talk about God's plans for those with a clean heart. Today, we're going to talk about the Holy Spirit's willingness to help us, because without the Holy Spirit involved in this process, we will end up focusing on the wrong things. We will rely on the wrong things, strive for the wrong things, and pray for the wrong things.

Have you ever felt helpless or ill-equipped for something? Maybe you feel that way with your fitness at times. Maybe it's with a parenting issue, school assignment, handyman project, or a job task. I mention those last four things because I've had firsthand experience struggling with all of them.

As a parent, I'm constantly challenged on how to rear our children to have grateful and submissive hearts.

Back in college, I had to take ancient Egyptian history. For my final, I had to write a paper on Queen Hatshepsut. Never heard of her? Neither had I. I was lost enough in this class as it was—a course that had no bearing on my writing degree whatsoever. (She was the first female Pharaoh, if you were wondering.)

About 10 years ago, a clogged sewer line backed up the plumbing at our old house. A smart homeowner would call for professional help. Instead, I thought I'd put my writing degree to use, which had no bearing on the plumbing issue whatsoever. I figured I'd snake the emergency overflow drain myself, measure the distance to the blockage, and dig a hole to fix the issue. I would have found China before finding the offending pipe.

Another time, I had the audacity to try and write a 90-day fitness devotional. I just wanted to guide people through the ups and downs of a fitness journey. I wanted to speak some truth into their lives in a brand-new way. I only wanted to reveal 90 profound and unique spiritual insights that could change their lives forever. I have a writing degree, after all!

In all four of these areas, I was and am ill-equipped. I have weaknesses. Here's the funny little secret: in relation to our heavenly Father, these aren't my only four areas of weakness. That's why I take great comfort in these verses:

> *"In the same way, the Spirit helps us in our weakness. We do not know what we ought to pray for, but the Spirit himself intercedes for us through wordless groans. And he who searches our hearts knows the mind of the Spirit, because the Spirit intercedes for God's people in accordance with the will of God."—Romans 8:26–27 (NIV)*

When Paul wrote this, he was undergoing great spiritual and physical suffering. If the Spirit can help Paul during the hardest of persecutions, can He not help us in our everyday lives? As The Living Bible puts it in verse 27, ". . . the Holy Spirit helps us with our daily problems and in our praying."

You see, right now, weeks 8–10 of this journey are arguably the hardest and can weaken us emotionally. As we're struggling with our "daily problems," we might earnestly seek Him. When we do, we often times unknowingly pray for the wrong things. We pray, "Lord, help me find time to work out" or the ever-popular "Father, help the numbers on the scale to go down."

Fortunately, I don't think that's what God hears. According to Romans, the Spirit searches our hearts and acts on our behalf. He takes our aching groans and makes our prayers presentable to our Father. Since the Father searches our hearts and knows the Spirit, God's will is orchestrated through His people.

Instead of "God, help me to be healthier," perhaps the Father hears, "Lord, help me rely on your Holy Spirit within me to be obedient to Your Word and bring You glory in all areas of my life."

Understand that our strength lies, in part, in acknowledging how weak we are. Then, in that weakness, the Holy Spirit works to empower us.

So keep approaching the God of all creation with your requests. Keep trusting that the Spirit is intervening on your behalf. There is great encouragement in this truth: in comparison to the perfect Holy Spirit, we are all weak; but, *by* the Holy Spirit, we are all strong!

Prayer

Father, thank You that in my weakness You are made strong. Will You forgive me when I underestimate the power of the Spirit? Please help me to rely on the promise that Your Holy Spirit is alongside me, helping, and prevailing. Amen.

Meditation

The Holy Spirit intercedes and empowers in my weakness.

Daily Spiritual Exercise

Today you are going to meditate for three to five minutes on Romans 8:26–27. Break each verse into its parts and pause to focus on what that means for your life.

For instance, in verse 26 we read, "… the Spirit helps us in our weakness." This means we are weak. We cannot do it on our own.

It also means we have the Spirit. Not only do we have the Spirit, our Spirit helps us in our weakness. Because of our weakness. Through our weakness. In spite of our weakness.

Furthermore, this means we are not alone. Not only that, but the one we are with, the one who lives in us, is able and is willing. How reassuring!

Proceed through the remaining passage in the same manner, applying these great promises to your life. When you're finished with verses 26–27, you can't help but to be more encouraged and empowered. In turn, verse 28 becomes not only more believable but more exhilarating:

> *"And we know that in all things God works for the good of those who love him, who have been called according to his purpose." (NIV)*

Week 8 Day 4 | *Promises in the Bible: All Things*

Kim grew up in a working-class family that made sacrifices to give her a private education. She excelled academically with a strong work ethic and an innate desire to do her best. She was a skilled volleyball player who was well liked by her peers. As a regular churchgoer, she had a religious background and she also had a grandmother who doted on her. It was a modest childhood, but a good one with many advantages others miss. Kim essentially walked the straight and narrow . . . until one day, she didn't.

At 15, Kim got pregnant. This was a shock to her friends and family and was devastating emotionally. "How could I, of all people, let this happen?" Battling through feelings of guilt, regret, and pain, she seemed to have a decision to make. Yet in her mind, there was never any question what she would do. She promptly ignored the advice of some of those around her. Then, at the ripe old age of 16, Kim gave birth to a beautiful, healthy son.

The story doesn't end there. With support from her family, she finished high school on time with a 4.0 GPA, while working a part-time job. She finished college early, with another 4.0 GPA; again, while working a part-time job and rearing her son. During this time, Kim realized that her "religious" background was not enough. Going to church was not enough. Believing in God wasn't enough. Certainly knowing the "right" answer was not enough. She decided she needed a personal relationship with her Creator. Then, for the first time, she truly surrendered her life to Christ.

After college, Kim was accepted into law school. However, she quickly recognized it would require too much time away from her son. She decided instead to go to graduate school part-time and get a master's in business administration. She had also been promoted a few times at her job at the bank. That led to being recruited for a position in the operations department of a trust company for a non-profit.

Around this time, Kim started dating a man who grew to love her unconditionally. He loved her not just in spite of her past, but, in part, because of it. After getting married and receiving her graduate degree, she was recruited again. This time she was going to run the operations department of a trust company with $2 billion in assets.

Fast-forward 10 years and three more children later, she is now a full-time mommy. She has volunteered as an encourager in a running group at her church. Kim gives regular talks there to single-moms who are facing what she once faced. Most recently, she helped start a crisis pregnancy center that helps people in unplanned pregnancies and post-abortive situations. They need love, support, and help where often none exists.

If you were to ask which is her favorite verse, Kim would quickly tell you:

"And we know that in all things God works for the good of those who love him, who have been called according to his purpose."
—Romans 8:28 (NIV)

There are several interesting things about this verse. First, it says, "in all things." Not in some things, or a few things, or in part of things, but in "all things."

We also see that "God works." He doesn't leave it solely up to us. He doesn't expect us to be the ones to do it all in our own power. Why? Because we can't! But He can and He wants to.

Also notice that He works "for the good of those who love him." That's us! He works for our good. For my good. For your good. For Kim's good. We are called to love Him with a pure heart and to follow His purposes for us. Then, He works on our behalf for our good. He works, but we benefit. What a deal!

Through the disapproving stares of strangers heaping shame on a pregnant teen, God worked! Through the incredible loss and torment experienced by Job, God worked! Through the adultery and murder by King David came Solomon. God worked! Through the death on the cross of His perfect Son, God worked! Through the countless failed diets, attempts to exercise, eating disorders, or lethargic lifestyle, God works! He works for our good for His purposes.

It's no wonder Romans 8:28 is Kim's favorite verse. It's no wonder why I married her.

Prayer

Father, thank You that nothing is wasted in my life, that You can use it all. Will You forgive me when I try to do the work. Will You forgive me when I don't trust Your purposes in my life? Please help me to always love You purely and completely. Amen.

Meditation

There is nothing that You can't work for my good.

Daily Spiritual Exercise

Meditate for three to five minutes on the promises found in Romans 8:28. As you think about "all things," narrow them down. One by one, lift up areas of your life that you need Him to work for your good. Nothing is off limits and there is no past issue that cannot be redeemed for His purposes.

Remember, nothing is wasted on God. He can use it all for His glory and our good. We are merely called to love Him and follow in obedience.

Week 8 Day 5 | *Promises in the Bible: He'll Provide*

Right now, you likely fall into one of three groups regarding this fitness journey.

For the first group, it's going great. They're seeing both physical and spiritual results. They're excited about the lifestyle changes they're making, and looking forward to continuing their progress after these 13 weeks.

If you're in the next group of people, you feel "okay" about the steps you've taken. However, you are the type that can do anything for a short period of time. It's what happens after these 13 weeks that concerns you. You're worried.

The final group of people are just hanging on by a thread. They may or may not be seeing results. They're having a hard time making anything feel like it will stick. If it's this hard now, what are the chances they'll survive after this fitness challenge is over? They, too, are worried.

The fizzle and fortitude phases of the journey claim many victims from these last two groups.

Bear with me. Examining nature might help.

Have you ever observed nature in action? I don't mean watching in passing, but actually paying attention. Squirrels are especially fun to spy on as they go about gathering acorns and burying their bounty for the winter. Zip-zap this way and that. They are frenzied but methodical, in a logical chaos we humans would not likely choose.

Take mighty ants, with a system opposite of the independent squirrel, marching in long lines of organizational perfection—an exercise in teamwork, with the efficiency and work ethic any military leader would be proud to command.

While squirrels and ants work differently, they share the commonality of an assured mindset. They prepare for tomorrow by only addressing today.

Heads down. Plow forth. "Now" is all we have.

You're thinking, "Of course they're not worried... it's nature. They don't know how to worry about the future." That's certainly true, and it's also the point. Worry is a learned behavior. It's also unproductive, even unbiblical. Worry presumes on things to come. Worry points to man's reliance on man to take care of the matter. Worry uncovers a lack of trust. Worry, at its root, is an act of disobedience. Fortunately, a look to Scripture is instructive and comforting.

Matthew 6 is loaded with common sense, making almost any argument in favor of worry look pretty silly:

> *"Look at the birds of the air; they do not sow or reap or store away in barns, and yet your heavenly Father feeds them. Are you not much more valuable than they?"–verse 26 (NIV)*

If God cares this much for the animals, how much more will He provide for us? I'll tell you. He sent His Son to die for us! In so doing, Christians are equipped for life on earth and are secured an eternity in heaven.

The very next verse is preeminent for those of us who value efficiency and productivity:

> *"Can any one of you by worrying add a single hour to your life?"*
> *—verse 27 (NIV)*

In other words, worry does you no good—of any kind at all—ever. It won't help you reach your goals. It won't foster a lifestyle of peace. Worry won't draw you closer to our Father. It only sucks life out of you.

In verse 33, we get to the crux of the worry issue: who are we looking to as our source of provision. Are we looking to our own efforts or to the efforts of our God?

> *"But seek first his kingdom and his righteousness, and all these things will be given to you as well."–(NIV)*

Unsurprisingly, the Bible has offered the perfect prescription against worry, and that's to seek Him first. When we do this, He'll provide for us both spiritually and physically.

Chapter 6 concludes with this gem:

"Therefore do not worry about tomorrow, for tomorrow will worry about itself. Each day has enough trouble of its own."—verse 34 (NIV)

Tomorrow already has a full plate; it doesn't need more. Tomorrow can do nothing for us in this moment. Yes, we have to plan, prepare, and pray for the future, but we are never to worry about it.

What's the difference? How do you know if it's worry or if you're just being prudent?

Worry produces ambiguity. Prudence produces a strategy.

Worry produces paralysis. Prudence produces action.

Worry produces doubt. Prudence produces confidence.

Worry benefits the devil, giving him a stronghold and fertile ground to plant seeds of doubt and discontent. Prudence honors the Lord, trusting in His provision as you go about obeying His commands.

The temptation to be worried about the future is the same even now, 2,000 years after Jesus was referencing the Gentiles in Matthew 6. We haven't changed. Worry is a byproduct of living on an imperfect earth; it's not a fruit of heaven. When we're consumed with things of this realm, we're not consumed with Christ, His kingdom or His righteousness.

What then does this mean for those who are prone to worry about their fitness future?

Heads down. Plow forth. Now is all we have, but Christ is all we need.

Prayer
Father, thank You for being the ultimate provider of my every need. Will You forgive me when I succumb to worry? Please help me to seek first Your kingdom and Your righteousness. Amen.

Meditation
You're my provider. Worry provides nothing but . . .

Daily Spiritual Exercise

Meditate on Matthew 6:26. If He cares this much about His creation, think how much He cares about you. After all, He sent His Son for you, not for the birds of the air.

As you meditate, think on how He has proven Himself faithful in your life. How He has loved on you. How He has provided for you.

When you do, you may end up feeling a little silly for ever fretting the future. For you have witnessed His trustworthiness time and time and time again.

Week 8 Day 6 | *Promises in the Bible: Iron Sharpens Iron*

My wife and I belong to a wonderful church with a senior pastor who is passionate about protecting and empowering families. When delivering a message regarding our children, he's fond of saying, "Show me their friends and I'll show you their future." Powerful and quite true. The companions our children choose will have no small impact on what kind of people they become.

The same can be said of us. According to personal development guru Jim Rohn, "You are the average of the five people you spend the most time with." Look at your five closest friends. There's a good chance you all share similarities, including wealth, faith, politics, and sports alliances. Even your fitness.

Before there was Jim Rohn, there was King Solomon. As we learned from Week 2, he was one wise dude. One of Solomon's most quoted verses is Proverbs 27:17:

> *"As iron sharpens iron, so one person sharpens another." (NIV)*

Friends can push you, challenge you, build into you, and shape who you are. Yet there are two facets about this verse that often go unexamined.

First, when a blade of iron is sharpened, it comes at the expense of iron shavings. Small fragments of the blade are scraped, ground, and lost. There's a cost for that iron and it may not feel so great. The same goes with your friendships. To be sharpened, you have to be open to a little pain at times. You have to be humble enough to acknowledge that parts of you must go. Making you into something stronger and more effective hurts a little.

The opposite of that verse also holds true: "As iron can dull iron, so one person can dull another." If the blade doing the "sharpening" is held at the wrong angle, it won't help. In fact, if the sharpening blade is rough and ridden with burs or laden with impurities, it will do more harm than good. The sharpening blade will shape the blade all right, just not in a way that will produce quality. The same will be true of you if you're not careful in your selection of friends.

That's why the right kind of accountability is so important when working on your fitness and making lifestyle changes. You need to be surrounded by people you respect and people who respect you. You need people in your life who are willing to say the hard things, but say them in love. You need people who want the best for you, people you wouldn't mind being like.

What kind of people are like that? Let's ask our buddy, Solomon. A friend loves at all times (Proverbs 17:17). A friend is reliably close (Proverbs 18:24). A friend's words have good intentions behind them (Proverbs 27:6). A friend's wisdom is sincere (Proverbs 27:9).

If that doesn't describe your friends, you must first ask, does it describe you? You attract what you exude. If you do have a friend like that, there's one more factor that will make all the difference, one thing that will increase the value of the friendship beyond measure.

Ecclesiastes 4:12 says, "Though one may be overpowered, two can defend themselves. A cord of three strands is not quickly broken." I would submit that the only third strand worth strengthening yourself by is our gracious God. When you have a friend who also shares a mutual dependence on God, the Holy Spirit is empowering you both. Remember, there's no limit to what God can do through His people.

If you're still struggling with your fitness, perhaps it's time to reach out to a true friend and ask for accountability. If you already have a friend supporting you, could you describe them the way Solomon does? Is God at the center of the friendship?

God puts people in our lives for many reasons. Allowing God to use them to make us more like Himself is one such reason. We would be wise to seek friendships that increase not just our happiness, but our holiness as well.

Prayer

Father, thank You that no matter what, You can be at the center of my support. Will You forgive me when I try to do it alone? Please direct me to people who love You more than anything else. Amen.

Meditation

Sharpen me that I might bring You glory.

Daily Spiritual Exercise

Proverbs is loaded with great verses regarding friendship. Read the following from Proverbs: 12:26, 17:17, 18:24, 27:6, 27:9, and 27:17.

After deciding which verse is your favorite, meditate on it for three to five minutes. Think about the implications the verse has for your life.

Thank God for the friendships He has given you.

Pray that you could be a friend to someone in need.

Pray also for wisdom regarding someone who could pour into you in a meaningful way, who could challenge you in your faith, who could help you grow in holiness.

Being sharpened may not be easy, but it sure beats being broken.

Week 8 Day 7 | *Promises in the Bible: Desires of Your Heart*

For a lot of people, certain things seem to come so naturally. Maybe these individuals are inherently charismatic, outgoing, and great with people. You, on the other hand, shy away from a crowd and have trouble connecting. Others might have the knack for knowing exactly what to do in a crisis situation. For you though, whether the incident is physical, spiritual, or emotional, you're more of a deer frozen in headlights. Do you have a close friend who is strong and decisive, able to make the right decision without hesitating? Not you. You fall victim to paralysis by analysis, debating for 30 minutes which shoes to wear with which dress or which plaid shirt to match with your jeans.

In instances like these, the temptation is to wish we were more like our friends. This results in praying that God would make us more like them or give us their personality traits.

We even cite Scripture to back up our appeals:

> *"Delight yourself in the LORD, and he will give you the desires of your heart."* —Psalm 37:4 (ESV)

The first problem with this is you're glossing over the fact that there's only one of you. In the entire history of this earth, there will ever only be one of you. That's it. No more.

He made you "you" for a reason. He has a plan for your personality. If you're busy wishing you were more like someone else, you're presuming you know better than He does. You are also failing to find your identity in Christ. Neither are good outcomes.

The next problem is that we forget the "delight yourself in the Lord" part. We pray and ask, but don't allow ourselves to be awestruck by our God. We aren't captivated by His creativity, fascinated by His faithfulness, or mesmerized by His magnificence. We don't stop to let Him "blow our minds."

Instead, we approach Him like a cosmic vending machine. We insert our prayer quarter. We make our selection for what we think we need in order to be what we think of as "happy." Then, we say "Amen" to collect our prize.

The heart wants what the heart wants. Besides, when we're happy, we can serve Him better, right? (Wink, wink.)

That leads us to the final issue. We fail to allow the "give" part of Psalm 37:4 to mean "provide," "put," or "place." In other words, letting God decide our desires for us and then place them in our hearts. We say we truly want what's best. We fully acknowledge that He knows better than we do. Being open to Him putting our wants on our hearts for us, rather than us putting them there, is difficult. If we did, we'd be more effective vessels. After all, when we're more effective living by, in, and for Him, we're inherently happier.

We are in the heart of the "fortitude phase" of this journey. As we trudge our way through the end of this week, you may be having some serious doubts. You can't see yourself ever waking up eager to get to your plyometric workout. You can't imagine a scenario resulting in you willingly ordering Brussels sprouts, sautéed in coconut oil and topped with walnuts. Certainly there will never be a time when you want to go to bed at a reasonable hour. Stressful days require de-stressing on the couch in front of the TV. You're questioning not only whether fitness will ever come effortlessly, but if you will ever even want it to come, effortlessly or not. It's work. It's hard. It's daunting.

What if we read Psalm 37:4 as "I will continually be amazed by You and I trust that You will change, align, and reorient my heart for Your purposes?" What if our hearts took a permanent posture of awe and wonder at what the Lord does? What if we trusted Him to take care of our desires for us? What do you think He'd want to do for and with a heart so submitted and respectful? My suspicion is plenty, including plenty with your fitness.

My challenge: don't pray that God would give you what you want. Pray instead that He would *make* you what He wants.

Don't be surprised later when the smell of sautéed Brussels sprouts makes you hungry.

Prayer

Father, thank You for Your endless delights. Will You forgive me when I want what You don't? Please help me to be concerned only with what You want for me. Amen.

Meditation

Let Your desires be my desires.

Daily Spiritual Exercise

Read Psalm 37:1–7a. When you're finished, pray that God would give you wisdom on how to apply this passage to your fitness.

After praying, go back to that same passage. This time, meditate on each verse, one at a time, for at least a minute. See if the Lord whispers something in you heart. It's okay if He doesn't, but I suspect He will.

When you're finished, pray that Psalm 37:4 would begin to characterize your life.

When we stay focused on delighting ourselves in Him, we can trust Him to take care of our desires and to use our personality for His purposes.

WEEK 9 PREVIEW

Running the Race

A race seems simple enough. Start digging a little, though, and you quickly find there's a lot to it. A race has different stages: start, middle, "the wall," and the finish. A race has many components: pacing, water breaks, the crowd, the racers, and the reward. Let's not forget the spectrum of emotions that come with it: uncertainty, excitement, nervousness, exhilaration, doubt, dread, and triumph.

That's why a race is the perfect analogy for what we're doing in our lives. Like a race, life requires a strategy. Float through it without intention and you'll find insignificance at the finish line. Just like a race, life is hard. Fighting the flesh might get easier, but it's never easy. A race is brief. In light of eternity, so are our lives.

This is why the New Testament uses the race analogy several times. It's easy for us to relate it to our Christianity. We see it in Acts, Galatians, 2 Timothy, Hebrews, and perhaps most notably in 1 Corinthians 9:24:

> *"Do you not know that in a race all the runners run, but only one gets the prize? Run in such a way as to get the prize." (NIV)*

The race Paul is referring to here, of course, is the Christian faith. Yet once again, we can also apply principles found in Scripture to our fitness. When we do, we find perfect instruction, conviction, and encouragement to guide us throughout this journey… a race in its own right.

Daily Spiritual Exercise: Read Scriptures aloud.
We are in the heart of the "fortitude phase" of Week 9. This might seem like a strange practice, but for your Scripture reading and prayers, talk to God out loud . . . not just in your heart. There's something about hearing yourself speak aloud that helps reinforce what you're actually saying. We need all the reinforcement we can get!

Week 9 Day 1 | *Running the Race: The Purpose*

Of the many components to a race, the one that most often goes unexamined is the purpose—more specifically, your purpose for participating. You might love group events, or you're the competitive type who loves a good challenge. If it's really intimidating, maybe you just want to prove to yourself that you have what it takes to finish. Or maybe you just like trying new things. There is no shortage of great reasons for doing a race.

In my case, the purpose was more insidious.

Years ago, my wife was bitten by the running bug and decided to do her first full marathon. She, unfortunately, ended up getting injured during her training. This was a bummer for a number of reasons. Of course, she was disappointed as she had trained so hard for so long. She was also sponsored to help raise money for a non-profit. Plus, the hotel reservation in Chicago was non-refundable.

So, I decided that if she couldn't run it, I would. I just couldn't bear the thought of the money for registration, sponsorship, and hotel going to waste. I trained the best I could in what time was remaining. On race day, I joined tens of thousands of others and didn't stop until I crossed the finish line. In fact, I did surprisingly well for someone who didn't like road running, especially road running for 26.2 miles.

A handful of years later, the feeling of being a "one-and-done" marathon hack was getting to me. I wondered how well I could do if I had a full 18 weeks of training. In my first marathon, I only had six. Thoughts crept into my head. "I have long legs. I can handle a fair amount of suffering before I quit. I'm reasonably disciplined. I bet I could qualify for Boston!" The running started up again and was going quite well . . . save for one small detail: I hated it. Remember, I don't like this sort of thing! It's long. Boring. Monotonous. Yuck.

Even still, I persisted with one thought propelling me: "It will be pretty impressive if, in only my second marathon ever, I qualify for Boston. I don't even like running!" That's a pathetic motivation that's hard to admit, but I'm being real.

Well, three weeks before the marathon, the Lord allowed me to have a hamstring injury. I couldn't race. All that training down the drain. All that dread the nights before long runs for naught. All my Boston-qualifying hopes dashed. To add insult to injury, wasted registration money. Ugh.

As Christians, the purpose for our fitness should be no different than the purpose for all areas of our lives: to honor God, to bring Him glory. This was certainly not the purpose for what would have been my second marathon. My purpose was my disgusting pride:

> *"Search me, O God, and know my heart; test my thoughts. Point out anything you find in me that makes you sad, and lead me along the path of everlasting life."—Psalm 139:23–24 (LB)*

For many people, pride is the purpose behind their fitness. Others might be motivated by guilt. Or influence. Or . . .

Of course, the Lord was gentle with me. In His loving way, He searched my heart, tested my thoughts, and pointed out where I was wrong. That conviction led me to not only ask for forgiveness, but to write about the experience here. Now, not only am I more aware and on guard against pride, He has allowed my example to teach others to do the same. He has taken an ugly situation and turned it around for His glory.

Don't misunderstand. There's nothing wrong with being pleased with the results of your fitness. Nor is there anything wrong with having fun racing. We just need to keep God at the forefront of our intentions. We need Him to test our thoughts and to lead our paths.

There's no better motivation for our fitness than pleasing our Father. Keep your purpose pure by keeping your eyes on Him.

Prayer

Father, thank You for your loving-kindness to me. Will You please forgive me for my pride? Please guide my thoughts, my heart, my path, and my purpose back to You. Amen.

Meditation

You are the purpose of my fitness.

Daily Spiritual Exercise

There are wonderful benefits for us when we take our fitness seriously. We look and feel better. We can serve and do more. We will likely live longer, more enjoyable lives. All great things. That said, the physical results we are hoping for with our fitness should not be synonymous with our purpose for it. Our purpose should be to glorify Him. The results are secondary.

Today, read Psalm 139 as a part of your out-loud Bible reading. As you hear yourself asking God to search your heart, listen to what He uncovers. Confess it to Him and pray for pure motives. Then rely on Him to direct and align your heart to His.

Week 9 Day 2 | *Running the Race: The Plan*

One of the many differences between novice and experienced runners is that novice runners "wing it." They train when they feel like it, if at all. They wear their lawn-mowing shoes and some cotton socks. The morning of the race, they're overdressed and under-hydrated. When the gun goes off, they start with a sprint and finish with a whimper.

Experienced runners know that running to win requires a plan. Their training is diligent, and it's specific. They do hill work, speed work, pace work, and long runs. Their equipment is individualized: shoes that match their foot type, with limited miles, worn with a synthetic blend sock. They understand that overdressing results in overheating, so they start the race cold. All week they've been hydrating. They know they'll lose pounds of water during the race, which if not replenished, will slow them down. When race day comes, they fight the impulse to give in to the adrenaline. Instead, they have planned the maximum pace they can maintain, while still finishing strong.

If we are to run to win, we will need a plan. Halfhearted efforts will give us halfhearted results. So winging it neither helps you nor honors God. We are called to do all things for God's glory:

> *"Don't you realize that in a race everyone runs, but only one person gets the prize? So run to win!"* – 1 Corinthians 9:24 (NLT)

Where winning our race toward fitness is concerned, we require a plan. A plan helps dictate performance. It gives us confidence and eliminates uncertainty. It gives us freedom because we are no longer enslaved to the nagging conviction of complacency and indifference. A plan gives us direction and hope as we finally have a roadmap to reach our goals.

Just like we don't fall into a good relationship with Christ, neither do we fall into being in good shape. We have to be intentional if we are going to see results. That intentionality requires a plan for our fitness, and our Father wants to be involved as we develop ours.

Here's the dirty little secret to a fitness plan: it changes. In fact, it must change as your health improves and your body develops. If there's an injury, if you get stronger or faster or lighter or heavier, adjustments need to be made.

Fitness plans also change when life "happens." Family schedules rearrange, new commitments are made, work responsibilities kick in, and vacations roll around. If you're struggling with a plan at Week 9 of this 13-week journey, hearing that change is inevitable should be a relief. Runners adjust their plans if they start to cramp or if they're running when it's especially windy. You can adjust your plan too.

That said, making an adjustment to your plan assumes you have one. You would not drive across the country without having a plan on how to get there. As 1 Corinthians 9:27 goes on to say, "Therefore I do not run like someone running aimlessly." We must take aim.

Having a hard time devising a plan? Pray for wisdom. God gives generously. If you have a realistic plan already, but are having trouble staying committed, pray for strength. God gives generously. Or if you're doing great on your plan, pray for continued endurance. God gives generously.

Relying on our God who gives generously to His children is always a good plan.

Prayer
Father, thank You that out of Your infinite wisdom, You can supply my needs in all areas of my life. Will You forgive me when I don't seek You or I don't run to win? Please bring balance to my plans that I might bring You glory at the finish line. Amen.

Meditation
God gives generously.

Daily Spiritual Exercise
As a part of your reading out loud today, include James 1, paying special attention to verses 5–8. These verses talk about wisdom and our need not only to pray for it, but to expect it. God, as verse 5 says, "gives generously." So pray that His generosity would be poured out over you, expect it, and praise Him when His wisdom comes.

Week 9 Day 3 | *Running the Race: The People*

If you've ever run or attended a large-scale marathon, you know just how great the people can be. Their encouragement rivals the camaraderie you share with strangers at baseball games. An unspoken trust occurs as you pass your hard-earned money down the row to the hot dog vendor. It's a rare moment as our collective selflessness provides a brief glimpse at what could have been, if not for our collective sinfulness.

Marathons are the same way. From the organizers and the volunteers, to the crowd and even the other racers, support is everywhere. Clangs of cowbells and random shouts of *"atta boy!"* Funny homemade T-shirts and witty signs. "Eye of the Tiger" blares on the loudspeakers, and children cheer from their parents' shoulders. It's a barrage of constant encouragement. It's why racers race . . . right?

Well, not exactly . . . at least not the sane ones. Yes, the people at the races can be inspiring and can give a well-needed boost when the event gets hard. Yet that's not why the runners are out there. The runners aren't running for the amusement of the crowd. They're mostly out there because of their own goals or dreams, to have fun or because they have a death wish. Whatever the reason, it's not to make the crowds or other racers happy.

Yet how often do we find ourselves working to impress others? How often do you catch yourself seeking approval from those around you, rather than from God? Our ugly pride can compromise the purpose for our fitness goals. Pride is also at the root of our intentions when we're performing for people as we run our races.

Nowhere in Scripture are we told that the purpose of obeying, pleasing, or working for man is *solely* for the sake of man. We ultimately do these things as unto the Lord. We want to reflect our faith in His purposes for our lives and bring Him glory.

For instance, we give "unto Caesar" not because we want to please our government. We do it because as Christ-followers, it pleases Him that we be law-abiding citizens. We aren't told to submit to one another so that we'll impress one another. We do it out of reverence for Christ.

Two different times Paul gives the same instructions to workers, once in Ephesians and again in Colossians:

"Whatever you do, work at it with all your heart, as working for the Lord, not for human masters . . ."—Colossians 3:23 (NIV)

Admittedly, this can be easier said than done—both the "all your heart" and the "for the Lord" parts. A lot of times it's one or the other. When we work for the Lord, however, we should want to work with all our heart. Conversely, we have to be on guard that when working with all our heart, we do so for the Lord.

This can get pretty tricky where our fitness is concerned. Even if we're authentically working with all our heart, we have to be careful. What begins as "for the Lord" winds up as "for men." What starts off as appreciating encouraging compliments regarding our progress quickly becomes the energy gels we feed on to keep us going. When this happens, we're running for "the people."

In Galatians 5:7, Paul says, "You were running a good race. Who cut in on you to keep you from obeying the truth?" Here he's explaining the freedom we have in Christ, as we live by the Spirit. This holds true for the fitness race you're running as well. Most of the people you're running with may be positive, well-meaning racers. However, a few will cut in on you and trip you up with their remarks: "You'll never lose that weight." "You'll always be scrawny." "Wow, you're ripped." These become the impetus for your running. Either "I'll show them" or "I'm a big deal" becomes your underlying mindset for your fitness. Without even realizing it, you're running not for the eyes of the Lord, but for "the people."

In the races we live, we'll always be running *with* people, but that's not the same as running *for* people. The good news is that God can help us recalibrate our motives. As Paul says to each of us in Colossians 3, "set your hearts on things above, where Christ is." We need to "set [our] mind on the things above…" We need to refocus our hearts and minds on Him. When we do, we take our eyes off the crowd. Off the racers. Off "the people."

If our primary purpose is to honor God with our fitness, then He should be the one on whom we are focused. Comments from outsiders, whether good or bad, should not be allowed to usurp His rightful place as our motivation.

Ultimately, we always win when we run for an audience of One.

Prayer

Father, thank You for allowing me to run for You. Will You forgive me when I look to people for my source of encouragement and motivation? Please help keep my mind set on You and You alone. Amen.

Meditation

You are the motivation for my fitness.

Daily Spiritual Exercise

Setting our minds on Christ is the best antidote to being negatively influenced by people. Of course, reading Scripture is a great way to align our minds to His.

Read Psalm 119 out loud as part of your reading today. This passage is an amazing reminder of God's faithfulness amid our struggles. As you do, ask the Lord that He and He alone would be the reason for your hope and comfort.

Week 9 Day 4 | *Running the Race: The Pace*

For those new to running races, the rookie mistake is to start too fast. And who can blame them? After 18 long weeks worth of training, it's finally race time. When the gun goes off, a gush of anticipation overwhelms them. All the pent-up nerves. The pre-race jitters. The flashbacks of smacking the snooze button before that 5:30 a.m. tempo run. The communal adrenaline spike from the thousands of other runners feeding off one another. It all results in an impulse to come out of the gate all-systems-go. The newbie thinks, "Why not capitalize on this burst of energy? I feel amazing."

At first, "amazing" sustains you. You're doing something you never thought possible. The crowd is cheering you on. Runners are still smiling. You look fantastic in all your running garb. At this speed, you'll crush your goal time.

Somewhere along the road, though, "amazing" betrays you… at mile four, or six, maybe mile eight, if you're lucky. Now you just feel "good." You think, "'Good' will do." And it does . . . until it doesn't. Then, "good" tags out for "okay," but "okay" doesn't last long either. "Okay" vacates to make room for "not great."

Soon you are feeling more bad than good. Eventually, the evil cousin of amazing—"miserable"—claims squatter's rights in your calves, quads, and hammies for the remainder of the race. If you finish at all, you swear off ever doing another race again. This downward spiral could have been avoided had you learned the fine art of pacing.

Throughout the Bible, we are trained with example after example on how to live the Christian life. Paul recaps a handful of them in Hebrews 11 and in 12:1. He implores us to use their examples to spur us on before giving us this sage advice on running:

> *". . . let us throw off everything that hinders and the sin that so easily entangles. And let us run with perseverance the race marked out for us, fixing our eyes on Jesus, the pioneer and perfecter of faith."*
> *—12:1b–2a (NIV)*

Sin hinders us. It trips us up and weighs us down. Strap a dumbbell to each foot and try to run. That is sin. Cast it aside, however, and you're more free not only to survive the race, but thrive in it.

As for our strategy, we have but one pace to run the race. It's not, however, so much a speed, such as fast, slow, moderate, or swift. Our pace is a mindset and that mindset is, as Paul tells us in Hebrews, "with perseverance."

Some translations say "endurance" and others say "patience." The point is we never give up. Races are long, hard, and grueling. Therefore, it's not about how fast we run, but about how we run . . . period. We should run with determination, purpose, and single-mindedness. Our pace is perseverance.

Keep in mind that although we're all running the same race, we all will have different routes. My race will look different than yours. Yours is different than your best friend's. Our goal, however, is the same: consistently surrendering our heart to God and following Him in obedience.

We can only do this, as we talked about yesterday, by setting our hearts and minds on things above. By "fixing our eyes on Jesus." Only He can direct our paths. Only He can supply our needs. Only He can perfect our faith.

There are two things that kill most people's fitness progress. The first is the inability to be honest with themselves about their efforts. The second is lack of perseverance. People start fast but burn out faster. They lack the determination to keep going no matter what. The truth is that most exercise and nutrition plans work for most people. People just quit the race too soon. People don't persevere.

However, when we adopt the mindset that our bodies do not truly belong to us (1 Corinthians 6:19), things change. Our goal becomes to consistently honor God with the body He gave us and trust Him with the results. We do this regardless of how slowly the mirror seems to change. We do this no matter how much change the bathroom scale reports to us. We do this no matter how good it feels, how fun it is, or how fast it happens.

When we commit to honoring God with our body no matter what, it is much easier to establish a healthy lifestyle. When we fix our eyes on Him, we no longer focus on the obstacles in the way. Or on the false timetables we create. Or on getting as fit as possible as quickly as possible. Fixing our eyes on Him enables us to persevere and to want to persevere.

If we trust Him with the race, we can trust Him with the pace.

Prayer

Father, thank You for Your promise to keep me going. Will You forgive me when I fail to run with perseverance? Please help me to be empowered by You and for You, that I might win the race You've designed for me. Amen.

Meditation

Only by You can I persevere.

Daily Spiritual Exercise

There is only one pace that produces a sustainably healthy lifestyle: perseverance. For the Christian, there is only one source that can sustain that perseverance.

Read Hebrews 11–12:3 out loud as part of your Bible reading for the day. You'll read example after example of the persevering faith of some of the Bible's greatest heroes.

As you read it, let it serve as a reminder that the gun has sounded. The race has started. If we are to run in such a way as to get the prize, we will have to persevere. Only He can empower us to run without growing weary . . . without losing heart.

Week 9 Day 5 | *Running the Race: "The Wall"*

Endurance athletes hit what is called "the wall" at one time or another. The wall is when your reserves of glycogen—the energy used for intense exercise—are almost depleted. The result is a sudden, total loss of energy. This kind of fatigue seemingly strikes you out of nowhere. When it does, it feels like you've run into a brick wall and can no longer go on. Everything feels heavier. Harder. Slower.

The wall isn't just what happens to you biologically. It's equal parts physical and emotional. When you hit it, your mind starts playing tricks on you. You hear the devil on your shoulder telling you that you can't go on. Making matters worse, you often hit the wall when you're about four-fifths through the race. Although there are many miles under your feet, the light at the end of the tunnel is still around several more corners. Over some hills. Through some shadeless long stretches and across some side streets. You are still far enough away from the finish line that the temptation to quit is both logical and justifiable.

Experienced athletes know there are ways to forestall the wall. The first step they take is to make sure their glycogen reserves are topped off before the race even begins. This is done by increasing the consumption of complex carbohydrates leading up to the race, which is known as "carb-loading." Secondly, taking in carbohydrates during the race will help replace some of what is spent during it.

The next thing they do to combat the wall is, of course, slow their pace. Lowering the intensity will cut down the amount of energy coming from glycogen. This gives them more mileage, but at a slower rate. Lastly, skilled runners are mentally equipped, knowing what to expect. This isn't only demonstrated by pre-race preparation and intra-race performance. Additionally, they are psychologically readied for the wall before it comes. They have an emotional game plan in place to combat the onslaught of negativity that floods the mind during the race's hardest stretch.

What's interesting about the wall is the mental aspects of it are not confined to athletic endeavors. You can hit the wall while working on reconciling your bank account, parenting the kids, or a long road trip. You can hit it while preparing for a final exam, cleaning the house, finishing a home improvement project, or writing a fitness devotional. You can hit it on most any long, drawn-out endeavor. Certainly, that includes a 90-day fitness journey. I've seen this not only in my own programs, but in most of the people I coach. When people hit the wall, they slow down, get discouraged, and want to give up.

What's also interesting about hitting the wall during a fitness journey is that it's mostly mental. At this point, completing the program is not an ability-based decision. After all, you've just demonstrated you can work out consistently or stick to the diet for nine weeks. It's now a character-based decision. Do you have the willingness, fortitude, and conviction to keep putting one foot in front of the other? To choose salads over chocolate. To choose yoga over TV. To go to bed early rather than surfing the web. Can you continue doing this day after day, but still taking it one day at a time?

As with the endurance athlete preparing to hit the wall, we can take similar precautions in this fitness journey. We do so not just to delay the wall, but knock it down altogether. By starting the journey with our spiritual tanks filled, we start the race fully equipped. In order not to run dry, we also are refilling our tanks every day, by prayer and by Scripture. We're mindful of God's ability to keep us going, knowing we've properly paced ourselves with perseverance from the beginning. Since we're focused spiritually, not just physically, we get the added benefit of His guidance mentally, as He renews our minds in Christ.

That's where it gets especially exciting for Christians. We don't have to rely on the character we were born with to determine if we will break through the wall. Instead, we can rely on the character we are *born again with*; the character of Christ in us can propel us forward. The character that gives us power and self-discipline (2 Timothy 1:7). The character that will complete the good work He began in us (Philippians 1:6). The character that will be with us always (Matthew 28:20). The very same character that enabled Paul to say confidently:

"I have fought the good fight, I have finished the race, I have kept the faith."—2 Timothy 4:7 (NIV)

Besides, God specializes in walls. He held up the walls of the Red Sea as Moses and the Israelites escaped the Egyptians. He tore down the walls of Jericho for Joshua's army. Through a hole in a wall, He saved the life of a reformed Saul. Then, by the sacrifice of His perfect Son, He destroyed the wall of sin that separates us from a perfect eternity.

When the wall hits, your response should really be no different from when you started this journey, or when you finish it. Check your motives. Align your will to His. Pray for His strength. Expect Him to give it. Praise Him when He does. Rely on Him solely. Give Him glory for working in your life.

Do this and you'll see something amazing: the walls you face in the race of life become the ways you grow in your walk with Christ.

Prayer
Father, thank You for the walls even though I don't always like them. Will You forgive me when my motives change, my will is misguided, or my strength is my own? Please help me to rely solely on You both now and when walls come. Amen.

Meditation
My walls are merely opportunities for God's strength to prevail.

Daily Spiritual Exercise
Read Philippians 1 out loud as part of your Bible reading today. Notice that Paul's chains, a wall in their own right, were used by God for His glory. Paul urged the church to "conduct yourselves in a manner worthy of the gospel of Christ." Amazing words coming from someone imprisoned for the very thing He is urging.

Setbacks in fitness, like those in life, are inevitable. Your responses to them will determine how quickly you recover. As a Christian, you can use these obstacles as reminders to check your purpose and your focus. Hitting a wall is really an opportunity to grow deeper in Christ.

Week 9 Day 6 | *Running the Race: The Breaks*

The general wisdom for running a race used to be simple: don't stop. The clock is running whether you're running or not, so until you cross the finish line, keep running.

The scientific knowledge in recent years has changed for all but the most elite runners. Studies show that walking one minute for every X minutes/miles you run can actually decrease your overall time, not increase it. Those brief rest periods give your muscles a much-needed break, letting them recover slightly in between the miles you're accumulating. It's also the ideal time to replenish lost fluids.

Rest periods give many people the ability to complete the race at a faster pace than would otherwise be possible. Rather than running on empty toward the finish line, you have some fuel in the tank to finish strong. Not only can you improve your run time, you'll enjoy the race more if you're not struggling throughout it. The same thing applies to your overall fitness plans.

When you engage in a fitness journey, especially when starting from scratch, periodic rest is needed. Rest keeps you healthy, injury-free, and consistently improving, and helps you enjoy the process. At least one rest day is needed each week, sometimes two or three.

Not all rest days are created equal. A day off may mean the complete absence of exercise, or it could be recovery-type workouts known as "active rest." These workouts are more focused on stretching, flexibility, breathing, mobility, and overall recovery. You're keeping your joints, muscles and ligaments loose, getting the blood flowing, and giving the body time to heal and refuel.

Your level of fitness and the intensity of the program you're doing determine how much recovery you need. Every four to six weeks, a full week of rest or active rest will be appropriate for most people. Your body can do some amazing things, but it just wasn't designed to go nonstop. Inadequate recovery leads to inadequate performance and results. Proper recovery, however, will improve your body's overall functioning with both your workouts and your day-to-day workload.

Rest breaks will also improve your spiritual conditioning. In fact, we need to refuel not just periodically, but daily. Spending time in the Word, in prayer, in praise, and in meditation with our Creator refuels us. We have examples to follow in the Bible that demonstrate this. David, a man after God's own heart, spent regular time with his Creator. Psalm 5:3 says, "In the morning, Lord, you hear my voice; in the morning I lay my requests before you and wait expectantly."

Daniel is another example from the Old Testament. He was in the daily habit of spending time with God. Daniel 6:10b says, "Three times a day he got down on his knees and prayed, giving thanks to his God, just as he had done before."

For the best example of how important it is to refuel spiritually, we once again turn to Jesus. God's own Son would often spend time alone with His Father and did so for a number of different reasons. He communed with the Father before choosing His apostles. Luke 6:12–13 tells us, "One of those days Jesus went out to a mountainside to pray, and spent the night praying to God. When morning came, he called his disciples to him and chose twelve of them, whom he also designated apostles."

He spent time alone with God both before and after performing miracles, such as in Matthew 14:23 and here in Mark 1:35, "Very early in the morning, while it was still dark, Jesus got up, left the house and went off to a solitary place, where he prayed." Because He was performing miracles often, He was frequently surrounded by crowds. Yet in spite of their needs, He prioritized time alone with God:

> *"But Jesus often withdrew to lonely places and prayed."*
> *—Luke 5:16 (NIV)*

Yes, Jesus was in constant communion with His Father wherever He went, but He also spent time alone with God. No crowds, no disciples, no apostles, and no family. If the Son of God needed time alone with His Father, how much more do we need it?

Time spent in the solitude of His presence is time we can get to know God and to hear from Him through His Word. We can't hear from Him if we're not spending time with Him. Not just that—think about how incredible it is that He wants to spend quality time with you. He wants to have you all to Himself. What a privilege!

Remember, to honor Him with our bodies we must first honor Him with our hearts. Doesn't matter if you call them "quiet times" or "Devotions." Doesn't matter if you do them in the morning or at night. Whatever combination of Bible reading, praying, singing, journaling, or meditating you choose, spending time alone with God needs to be a non-negotiable, daily activity. They're just like rest days in an exercise program, walk breaks in a marathon, or sleep at night. They'll help you function better, grow spiritually, and enjoy the blessing of His regular presence in your life.

Finishing strong requires refueling often. There's no better rest break than one spent with the only One who can truly renew your strength.

> *"But those who hope in the Lord will renew their strength. They will soar on wings like eagles; they will run and not grow weary, they will walk and not be faint."—Isaiah 40:31 (NIV)*

Prayer
Father, thank You for wanting to spend time with me. Will You forgive me when I choose something or someone else over a rest break with You? Please help me develop a deep affection for the time we spend together. Amen.

Meditation
My breaks with You help me finish strong.

Daily Spiritual Exercise
Physical rest is not only needed, it's not only healthy, but it's biblical.

Today, read aloud Isaiah 40. As you do, you will be reminded that spiritual rest, communing with the Father and being still, is not only needed, it's not only healthy, it's not only biblical, but it's a gift. Time alone with our God is a gift that satisfies, refuels, and rejuvenates the soul. A gift that equips you to honor your Creator. A gift that enables you to persevere in the race.

Week 9 Day 7 | *Running the Race: The Finish*

An avid racer will tell you that there's a big difference between finishing and finishing strong. Somebody who merely finishes might only feel relief, exhaustion, or even disappointment. Strong finishers, however, while still tired, feel pride, accomplishment, and satisfaction knowing that they executed to the best of their ability. Whatever positive feelings "mere finishers" have are born out of the removal of something negative. Strong finishers' feelings stem from the achievement of something positive. Though the race was hard, they did all they could, the best they could, for as long as they could and powered through the finish line.

As we've talked about this week, our fitness is its own kind of race. Body stewardship is a funny thing. Whereas other kinds of stewardship might get easier as we get older, fitness... not so much. For instance, as we enter retirement, we're not likely to start blowing all of our money on pointless pursuits. We know our bank accounts need to outlast us. We will be wise with our money. As we get older, we also realize more and more the value of our relationships, especially with our families. So, we look for ways to spend more time with them. We will be intentional with the time we have remaining.

Yet with fitness, our bodies are working against us. Not only does exercise get harder, the basic physical routine of life gets harder. Our sleep might increase, but so does our waistline. It's a deadly combination of a less active lifestyle and a greater temptation to use food as entertainment. You may not be able to run as far or as fast; but, hey, you can always eat out, right? Then the cycle of a more sedentary life and a focus on food perpetuates itself, each feeding on the other. Although other areas of stewardship might improve, finishing strong with our fitness gets more and more challenging. Challenging, but not impossible.

For the model on finishing strong, we once again turn to the Apostle Paul. Paul set a wonderful example for us on how to run a race: he was intentional with every factor. He had a clear *purpose* for the race: complete the task Jesus gave him of sharing the good news (Acts 20:24). His *plan* was to do all he could to build an effective and upright church body, ensuring that his work was not in vain (Philippians 2:16). His *pace* was perseverance, as he kept the faith and fought the good fight (2 Timothy 4:7). Neither *people* nor *walls* could stop him because he would just turn them into *breaks* that refueled him (Acts 16:25–40).

For Paul, finishing strong included being martyred for his faith. My guess is in those final moments he had only one thing on his mind. He wanted to receive the heavenly prize for which he had been called (Philippians 3:14).

For Paul, the race was hard. Yet he did all he could, the best he could, for as long as he could.

I believe that fitness, for Christians, is a reflection of or a response to their faith. Similar to our faith, strong fitness requires doing the hard things in the hard times. Strong fitness takes effort. It doesn't happen overnight. It's a process. Not unlike faith, one needs to "work out their fitness with fear and trembling" (Philippians 2:12). Just like with our salvation, as Paul goes on to say, He will work in us:

> *". . . for it is God who works in you to will and to act in order to fulfill his good purpose."—Philippians 2:13 (NIV)*

Paul understood God was at work in him to accomplish God's will. Paul must have desperately held on to this promise up through the time of his death. You see, Paul was never the one doing the work. He was not "willing" his way to the finish line. He was never the one "acting." Paul was never the one fulfilling the purpose. God was at work. It was God working through Paul to accomplish His purpose for Paul and for God's greater good. Paul finished the race strong because God carried him through.

God will carry you, too, if you let Him. We are all in the fitness race. We will all finish the fitness race. We will not all finish strong however. The degree to which we rely on God "to will and act in order to fulfill His purpose" determines how strong we finish. Our reliance on Him also dictates how much we enjoy the run.

In the 1981 Academy Award–winning movie *Chariots of Fire*, there's a great scene with one of the protagonists, Eric Liddell. Eric, a devout Christian and Olympic hopeful, is confronted by his sister for missing a prayer meeting. Though she questions his faith, Eric tells her that he intends to someday return to the mission field in China. Now though, he feels he needs to focus on running, "I believe that God made me for China. But He also made me fast, and when I run, I feel His pleasure."

God made each one of us for a purpose . . . for His purposes. That purpose includes involving Him to empower us. If we go the road alone, trying to operate out of our strength, we will merely finish.

When we rely on Him in us, however, we too will feel His pleasure. It strengthens us to do all we can . . . the best we can . . . for as long as we can. It strengthens us to finish strong.

Prayer
Father, thank You for getting me this far. Will You please forgive me when I complain about the journey? Please help me to always rely on You in me, so that I might feel your pleasure. Amen.

Meditation
You finish strong in me.

Daily Spiritual Exercise
Read 1 Corinthians 9:24–27 as part of your Bible reading today. Then, as you're praying out loud, ask God for His strength to work in you, not just for your fitness but in your faith. God works in us to finish what He starts.

Tell Him you don't want to merely finish. Ask Him to empower you that you might run in such a way to get the prize and fulfill His good purpose.

The Lord Is _____

How would you fill in the blank above? On one hand, it's really easy because He is so many things. There is no shortage of adjectives that apply to our Lord.

On the other hand, where do we begin? I mean how do we adequately describe the One who is the Lord of all the Earth? There aren't enough books to contain descriptions of our Lord and His love for us.

Frederick M. Lehman wrote in the great hymn, "The Love of God":

> *Could we with ink the ocean fill,*
> > *And were the skies of parchment made,*
> *Were every stalk on earth a quill,*
> > *And every man a scribe by trade,*
> *To write the love of God above,*
> > *Would drain the ocean dry.*
> *Nor could the scroll contain the whole,*
> > *Though stretched from sky to sky.*

Here's the thing: even though we can't adequately describe Him, He's still honored when we try.

If my six-year-old daughter were asked to describe me and she wrote, "Daddy takes care of me," or "My daddy helps me when I'm scared," her words would melt my heart. Not because those illustrations completely describe me and all that I do for her as a parent. They fall far short of that. Her words honor me by giving me a peek into her heart and what I mean to her. Her descriptions also help me see that she understands, on some small level, how valuable she is to me, how much I cherish taking care of her and being her father.

We are in Week 10 of this fitness journey, still persevering through the fortitude phase. Now, more than ever, we need to seek the Lord. We need to better understand who He is and to acknowledge how important He is to us. Then, when we dive deep into who the Lord is, we start to see how important we are to Him!

Over the course of this week, we will examine what Scripture says about who the Lord is. We will look at some of the more popular conceptions about the Lord. We'll also see some of the less obvious ideas about who the Lord is—ones that aren't the first words to pop into our heads when thinking about filling in that blank. We'll find that both the common and less common descriptors equip us to battle our way through the week. At the end of the week, we'll have emerged victorious because, well, our Daddy takes care of us too.

Daily Spiritual Exercise: Write a prayer of praise.
Every day this week take 10 to 15 minutes to examine one adjective you would use to complete the sentence, "The Lord is_____." Take a closer look at how just one of the attributes of the Lord has empowered, comforted, or sustained you. By working on it a little each day, you'll have written a love letter to the Lord by week's end.

Don't worry about being profound or eloquent. That's not the goal. It's about recognizing the Lord's character and paying Him the honor He deserves. This will likely be the most challenging daily spiritual exercise you'll do during our fitness journey . . . and potentially the most rewarding.

Week 10 Day 1 | *The Lord Is: My Banner*

It's hard to sing "The Star-Spangled Banner" and not envision the epic battle that took place at Fort McHenry in 1814. We can almost see the weapons being fired. We can nearly feel the earth shake as the bombs explode. We can just about smell the stench of smoke and gunpowder. By song's end, our pride swells, as a tattered American flag still stands tall, waving in the wind.

A country's banner (or flag) should elicit pride in the heart of its citizens. For the United States, Old Glory represents sacrifices made by our brave military to preserve the liberties we hold dear. Our flag represents the 50 states formed from the 13 colonies that first declared independence from Great Britain. She represents strength, legacy, dignity, and home. It's meant to be flown high, on display as a sign of respect for the fallen—a symbol of gratitude for our freedom.

Yet as much as our flag means to us, neither she, nor anything or anyone else, should be our personal banner. Our banner is the Lord. This is something Moses understood quite well.

In Exodus 17, we read about an interesting fight between Joshua and the Amalekites. Joshua had engaged the Amalekites, as Moses had instructed. Joshua was winning, but only when Moses' hands were held up in the air. As soon as Moses dropped them, the Amalekites would have the advantage. Moses kept his hands up, but as you can imagine, his arms would get tired. Moses received help from Aaron and Hur, one on each side, to keep his hands high until sunset. Finally, Joshua overcame the enemy. Then we read:

> *"Moses built an altar and called it The Lord is my Banner."*
> *—verse 15 (NIV)*

Moses understood where the victory came from and who should receive credit. Moses didn't give Joshua the victory. There certainly wasn't anything magical about Moses' hands. Nor would Joshua or any of his fallen soldiers get the credit. In fact, neither did national or ethnic pride. After all, Moses didn't name the altar "Israel is my Banner." The Lord and the Lord only gave the victory.

Well, the Lord is my banner too . . . and He's yours. He's the banner of all who have professed Jesus as the Son of the Living God and as their personal Savior. Not unlike an American banner, the Lord as our banner represents many things for us. With only a few weeks left in this 13-week journey, remembering who gives the victories is of utmost importance.

First, our banner represents what has already been done. The war over sin and death has already been won. The Lord already sent his Son. The ultimate victor has declared the ultimate victory.

Now you still may have struggles with food, lethargy, or addictive be-haviors. Pride, balance, or physical ailments might be tripping you up. It's important to keep in mind that while these are very real battles, the outcome has already been decided. Yes, you're still in the battlefield. Yes, Satan is still firing mortars at you. And yet he's still on the losing side, no matter how frightening the battle becomes.

Second, if the Lord is our Banner, and our Banner is in charge of our lives, should we not feel emboldened? If the Lord is Lord over all and truly the Lord of our lives, is there anything we have to fear? Is there any battle too big? Any fight too fierce? If He has claimed the biggest victory there is to claim, can He not also win the smallest? Of course He can!

Those struggles you might still be facing? He can still win! It's not over. They are winnable skirmishes in an already won war.

Third, a banner is meant to be on display. It's meant for people to see. It's meant to be recognized and understood as a symbol for something greater. The Lord is that "something greater." In fact, He is the greatest and no one else even comes close.

As our banner, we give the Lord credit for whatever success we have with our fitness. We need to fly His name high as the motive, power, and giver of our progress—whether you've lost a lot of weight or a little, or whether you exercised regularly or on occasion. Whether sleep has improved or stayed the same, He has sustained you over these weeks. He has kept your arms lifted and will continue to do so. As such, we should take a cue from Psalm 20:5, which says, "May we shout for joy over your victory and lift up our banners in the name of our God."

Moses had it right: the Lord is our banner. God is the symbol and giver of victory. He's worthy of all the praise and glory and honor, doing for us what we can't do on our own.

With the Lord as our banner, we remember not only what He has done, but we also have confidence in what He can continue to do. This includes what He can do with our fitness. Then, as He works our good for His glory, we need to remember to give Him the praise He deserves.

Prayer
Father, thank You for being both the symbol and giver of victory. Will You forgive me when I lose perspective or lose hope in what You have already done? Please help me to unabashedly give You the praise and glory for what You are doing in my life. Amen.

Meditation
The Lord is my banner.

Daily Spiritual Exercise
Spend 10 to 15 minutes writing your own "The Lord is_____" devotional prayer of praise. Remember, you don't need to be eloquent to honor God by this exercise. The goal is to acknowledge who He has been, is, and will continue to be in your life. Don't get caught up in making it perfect. It's the pouring out of your heart that brings Him glory.

Week 10 Day 2 | *The Lord Is: Good*

"Good" is such a generic term. "This chicken tastes good." "That was a good movie." "How are you doing? Good." What a boring adjective that more often than not does a poor job of actually describing the subject you're discussing. The chicken might be good, but compared to what? Tuna? Did you mean it was flavorful and juicy? Was it good in the sense that it's better than nothing . . . it's fine . . . it will do?

What then do we make of this popular verse in Psalm 106:1, 1 Chronicles 16:34, Ezra 3:11, Psalms 117, 118, and 136?

> *"Give thanks to the Lord, for he is good; his love endures forever."*
> *—Psalm 106:1 (NIV)*

Yes, He is good, but good compared to what? Other gods? Well, yes, of course.

He's good in that He is full of life and hope? Yep.

He's good compared to the absence of a god? Well, that, too, but so much more.

The Bible actually tell us just how good He is. You see, nearly every time it refers to the Lord as "good," it follows with "his love endures forever." So, the Lord is faithful, persistent, sustaining, everlasting, and perfect. Do you know of anyone else whose love is this way?

A few years back when our youngest was born, I emailed the men in my Bible study group the news:

"Silas William Pryor was born at 6:20 p.m. weighing 9 pounds 1 ounce, 22 inches long. Mommy is doing great. Thanks for the prayers."

The responses were all congratulatory and happy for the safe delivery. "Congrats!" "Way to go, Mom!" "Happy for you, brother—God is good." However, for the first time, the common response of "God is good" struck me differently.

Yes, yes, God is good. A healthy baby is what we prayed for and He graciously gave a perfectly healthy son.

Yet even if Silas had been born blind, deaf, or crippled, it wouldn't diminish God's goodness. In fact, His goodness can't be diminished . . . only magnified. Why? Because His love endures forever. His goodness, his enduring love would have sustained us throughout Silas' life. This is true whether Silas were born healthy or born with a crippling deformity or genetic disease. Through the tears of heartbreak, God's love would endure. Through the silence of unanswered questions, His love would endure. Through limited mobility at the park when the other children were running freely, His love would endure. Through the special education or physical therapy he would require, God's love would endure. There's no end to something that endures forever! Then, as we became more like Jesus during the very trying times, His goodness would be all the more magnified.

It's hard not to be comforted by this. His love is so good that it will sustain us not just with our fitness, but in all areas of our lives. As His love propels us, we will be able to recognize Him as the source of our strength. We will, as the verse declares, "Give thanks to the Lord," and watch as His goodness is magnified!

While we're on the subject of giving thanks, notice that the verse isn't really presenting love and thankfulness as an if/then statement. The verse is not saying that thankfulness is an option either. The verse is not saying, "If his love endures, give thanks." Nor is it saying, "Because of his love, if you'd like to, you can give thanks." In fact, the "give thanks" comes first. We give thanks ahead of time. This is an important distinction. Otherwise, we're tempted to proclaim God's goodness only in the times of blessing, as when Silas was born healthy. What then will we do during times of trial, such as when we later learned Silas had a life-threatening food allergy?

As for your fitness, give thanks for it. Give thanks whether your results have been amazing or abysmal, for God is good. From His goodness, He can sustain your continued efforts that you might in turn bring glory back to Him.

You see, things are much different when you understand that the end of the story has already been determined. It's much easier to rest, rejoice, and give thanks knowing His love prevails regardless of how hard the situation might be. His love is from everlasting to everlasting.

If the measure of "good" is a love that endures forever, then that description is good enough for me.

Prayer
Father, thank You for the miracle of Your everlasting love. Will You forgive me when I gloss over the depths of Your goodness? I pray that in all areas of my life, Your goodness, Your enduring love, would be magnified. Amen.

Meditation
You are good in all things, for all times.

Daily Spiritual Exercise
Continue to spend 10 to 15 minutes writing your own "The Lord is_____" devotional prayer of praise. Remember, you don't need to be eloquent to honor God by this exercise. The goal is to acknowledge who He has been, is, and will continue to be in your life. Don't get caught up in making it perfect. It's the pouring out of your heart that brings Him glory.

Week 10 Day 3 | *The Lord Is: Close*

A few years back, I was in Tanzania with Here's Life Africa. It's an amazing ministry that takes the gospel out into the bush to evangelize and disciple the wonderful people of Africa. Now, the distance from Louisville (where I live) to Arusha (where we stayed) is about 8,100 miles.

For a little context, that's a little less than driving from the East Coast of the United States to the West Coast, then back to the East Coast, then one more time to the West Coast again. The journey required several long flights to arrive half a world away. Another world it was . . . new sights, sounds, tastes, and smells. While our hotel had modern accommodations and the people were welcoming, I felt very, very far from home.

At night, I was able to call my family. In that moment, I was instantly transported back to a very familiar, very comfortable place. Hearing the voices of my wife and children transported me. I felt the coziness of our house. I could see them in my mind's eye. I could hear the love in their hearts. While it seemed I was on a different planet, I felt close.

This, to me, is similar to how our relationship to the Lord sometimes feels. While at times it might seem like He's on a different planet, He's as close as a conversation. Actually, if He lives in our hearts, by definition He's closer to us than anyone else possibly could be.

Admittedly, it can be hard to feel close to someone we talk to but who doesn't answer us audibly. Someone we've never seen face to face. Someone we've never touched with our own hands.

However, we have assurances in Scripture that He is indeed with us wherever we are:

> *"The righteous cry out, and the Lord hears them; he delivers them from all their troubles. The Lord is close to the brokenhearted and saves those who are crushed in spirit."—Psalm 34:17–18 (NIV)*

We see His closeness displayed again later in Psalm 145:

> *"The Lord is near to all who call on him, to all who call on him in truth. He fulfills the desires of those who fear him; he hears their cry and saves them."—verses 18–19 (NIV)*

Then again, we see His closeness in the New Testament:

> *"Let your gentleness be evident to all. The Lord is near. Do not be anxious about anything, but in every situation, by prayer and petition, with thanksgiving, present your requests to God. And the peace of God, which transcends all understanding, will guard your hearts and your minds in Christ Jesus."—Philippians 4:5–7 (NIV)*

We are nearing the end of what's arguably the hardest phase of the fitness journey, the fortitude phase. Success in this phase is often nothing more than showing up. Put one foot in front of the other, focus on the behaviors, and trust that the physical results will follow.

That's why recognizing just how close the Lord is to us is such an enormous help. It's like having running partners. They cheer us on, hand us water and energy gels, match us stride for stride, even hold our hand if necessary.

Yet our Lord is even closer than that. What's especially encouraging is the outcome of His closeness. It's what happens when you "cry out," "call on," relinquish anxiety and prayerfully "present your requests" to God.

He doesn't stop at just being close to us. Look back at each of the verses and you see He's at work. He "delivers," "saves," "hears," "fulfills," "saves" some more, and "guards" our hearts and minds!

While the Lord may feel a million miles away, the Bible makes it clear that He is close to you. He hears you when you pray, so pray. He hears you when you call, so call. He hears you when you cry out, so cry out. As you do, remember, after He listens, He supplies your needs.

So, call out to Him because He's as close as a conversation.

Prayer

Father, thank You for not only being close, but delivering me in so many ways. Will You forgive me when I seek deliverance from anyone other than You? Please help me to better rely on who You are and what You are able to do through me. Amen.

Meditation

The Lord is close . . . and able.

Daily Spiritual Exercise

Continue to spend 10 to 15 minutes writing your own "The Lord is____" devotional prayer of praise. Remember, you don't need to be eloquent to honor God by this exercise. The goal is to acknowledge who He has been, is, and will continue to be in your life. Don't get caught up in making it perfect. It's the pouring out of your heart that brings Him glory.

Week 10 Day 4 | *The Lord Is: Trustworthy*

It's always exciting to see people make a public declaration of faith and then follow in obedience by being baptized. At our church, when Christians are baptized, they recite something called "The Good Confession." It goes something like this: "I believe that Jesus is the Christ, the Son of the Living God, and I trust Him as my Lord and Savior." The person making that confession is then immersed in water, representing the death, burial, and resurrection we have in Christ.

What a humbling and powerful admission to make. However, have you stopped to consider what "trust as" means? It signifies that we are turning over everything to Him. Jesus is Lord of all, and as such, He can take care of us, the entire us.

Sometimes, though, we unknowingly differentiate between "trusting God as" and "trusting God with." This is a distinction without a difference, yet that's not how we treat it.

Have you ever tried teaching a child how to jump into a swimming pool? With both of my girls, the process was pretty much the same. They had plenty of experience playing in a pool. However, standing on the edge—with the prospect of throwing themselves in the air—presented a new challenge. With my hands outstretched, willing and waiting, I would say, "Do you trust me to catch you?" They would always say yes.

They knew I was more than capable, as they had certainly seen me carry things much heavier than they were. They'd also seen me navigate the waters without issue. Furthermore, I've always been sure to keep my promises in the past. They said that they trusted me "as" their daddy to catch them, yet they still couldn't quite bring themselves to jump. It was safe to assume that some part of them somewhere didn't trust me "with" their complete safety.

If we're not careful, the Christian life looks a lot like the child on the edge of the pool. We know in our heads that God is God. He's the maker of heaven and earth, conqueror of death, and giver of eternal life. Yet, when push comes to shove, our hearts are reluctant to completely relinquish some parts of our lives. Maybe it's unintentional. It just never occurs to us to turn over every part of our life to the Lord. Or perhaps we question as to whether He even cares about the "little stuff."

However, the Lord doesn't want us only to trust Him "as" the Lord of our lives, our Savior from death. He wants us to trust Him "with" our lives, for He is the Giver of life, both on earth and for eternity. There should be nothing in our lives that is off-limits to the Lord, including our fitness.

Just look at the encouragement we have in the Book of Psalms:

> *"The Lord is trustworthy in all he promises and faithful in all he does."—145:13 (NIV)*

This means in everything He does, God is trustworthy. If we involve Him in our fitness, we have the assurance of His faithfulness.

How do we involve God? Every day we turn our fitness over to Him. We "give" the Lord both our struggles and our victories. We praise Him no matter what. We look for ways to grow deeper in our relationship with our Father. We acknowledge that lasting good will only come out of our fitness if we trust Him "with" it.

Please don't confuse His trustworthiness and faithfulness to mean that He will always answer your prayer the way you want. You might shed fat; you might not. You might run faster; you might not. You might become stronger; you might not.

What we can be assured of is that when we trust in Him, we will not be shaken (Psalm 125:1). We know that He has a plan and is working that plan for our good (Romans 8:28). He has compassion for us (Psalm 145:9). He will sustain us amid our defeat (Psalm 145:14). He has it all under control (Psalm 145:15). Most importantly, if He's involved, He will be glorified in it (Psalm 145:10).

If you aren't as close to reaching the results as you had hoped, this might be the hardest phase of the fitness journey. You may have worked hard and sacrificed a lot for what seems like little in return. This disappointment is only compounded when you realize that you might not be fully trusting Him.

Persevere. Trust God not only "as" your Savior but "with" every part of your life. God is strong and able. He is deserving of being trusted as our Lord. He is worthy of being trusted with our fitness efforts.

When you don't think you can stick to your exercise program, trust your Father to sustain you. When Satan temps you to turn to food for comfort, trust the Lord to deliver you. When your fitness ambitions are motivated by what people think rather than by what the Lord says, trust that God can change you. When you're paralyzed by a lifetime of a poor body image and emotional wounds, trust the Great Physician to heal you. Turn over your fitness completely to the Lord and see what He will do with it.

No more standing on the edge of the pool. No more debating whether you can do it. No more waffling as to whether or not God will catch you.

He is standing with His hands outstretched, willing, and waiting. Jump!

Prayer
Father, thank You for being trustworthy with all areas of our lives. Will You forgive me when I hold back part of my heart? Help me to recognize when I'm operating out of my trust in myself. Help me then turn it over to Your very capable hands. Amen.

Meditation
I trust You as my Savior and with my life.

Daily Spiritual Exercise
Continue to spend 10 to 15 minutes writing your own "The Lord is_____" devotional prayer of praise. Remember, you don't need to be eloquent to honor God by this exercise. The goal is to acknowledge who He has been, is, and will continue to be in your life. Don't get caught up in making it perfect. It's the pouring out of your heart that brings Him glory.

Week 10 Day 5 | *The Lord is: Faithful*

While I'd certainly like to, I doubt I'll ever forget that Christmas Eve. Not old enough to be in school, I was still in my "Christmas is magic" prime. We weren't taught about Santa. Yet the way my parents made Christmas so special, we didn't need that dude. We had Christmas enchantment all season long.

Mom had slaved over the decorations, festivities, and traditions all December long. She and Dad were talking about something in the kitchen. However, the unwrapped presents—the last remaining task on their to-do list—were lurking in the basement. With my brothers upstairs and parents distracted, the temptation to steal a peek at the bounty was just too much.

So, down the stairs I crept to take a gander at the spread, and what a beautiful spread it was! Surely it would be the best Christmas ever, if it had not wound up being the worst. I stealthily exited the premises undetected. In my enthusiasm of the successful mission, I somehow disclosed too much "intel" to one of my brothers. My supposed comrade-in-arms turned on me and promptly ratted on me to the authorities. A hearing quickly convened and disciplinary action ensued.

Temptation is everywhere, all the time, no matter what. It's the primary instrument of marketers, bombarding us with sights and sounds that sow seeds of discontent. It's the magnetic tug of our sinful nature. Temptation pulls us into harm's way, pushing us against the direction we're trying to travel, like running into the wind. It's Satan's native language. He whispers lies, half-truths, distortions, and doubts in our ears, often times without us knowing, every time in an effort to kill, steal, and destroy.

Temptation in the conventional sense overcame some popular figures in Scripture: Adam and Eve, Samson, and David. Temptation is at the root of every sin. Sin stains everyone in the Bible—everyone except our Jesus.

That said, we have some great examples of people who overcame temptation: Job, Joseph, David, Peter, John, Paul, and Silas.

At the core of all of their victories in the face of temptation was their reliance on the Lord's faithfulness. The Lord had previously been faithful to these men. In their moments of crisis, these men expected the Lord to remain so. Jesus Himself held fast to His Father's faithfulness. The Father's faithfulness supplied what Jesus needed, while Jesus supplied what the world needed.

We have many wonderful verses to remind us of the Lord's faithfulness. One of the most helpful is found in the New Testament:

> *"The temptations in your life are no different from what others experience. And God is faithful. He will not allow the temptation to be more than you can stand. When you are tempted, he will show you a way out so that you can endure."—1 Corinthians 10:13 (NLT)*

What we face is ultimately no different than what others have faced; it's just wrapped in a different package. That fateful Christmas at the age of four . . . the temptation I succumbed to . . . is really no different than the trials I face at the age of 41. It's just that now the presents are different.

What's exciting is that God's faithfulness is no different. It's the same now as it was 37 years ago . . . as it was 2,000 years ago. Out of the Lord's faithfulness to us, He will both empathize with us (Hebrews 4:15) and empower us to escape from looming disaster (Hebrews 4:16).

The temptation to question, compromise, give up, not start, blow off, or put off your fitness convictions will likely never stop. Why would it subside, if Satan came to kill, steal, and destroy?

Yet out of God's great love, He sent Christ to save us. He sent Christ to heal us. He sent Christ to give us life and life to the full. The saving, healing, giving life of God's faithfulness will be more than enough provision. It will deliver us in our greatest times of need. This is true for a preschooler on the verge of ruining Christmas for himself. This is true for adults on the verge of giving up on their health.

The Lord has only ever been faithful. It would then make sense that He will continue to be so. Surrendering your fitness to Him and trusting Him with the results will strengthen your faith and glorify Him in the process.

So, never, ever forget . . . God is faithful. There is no temptation that will be more than you can stand, when you're standing with Him.

Prayer

Father, thank You for being faithful to me. Will You forgive me when I fail to recognize Your sustaining grace and mercy? Please help me to hold onto the truth of who You are. You've displayed that throughout not just my life, but throughout the ages. Amen.

Meditation

The Lord is faithful and willing.

Daily Spiritual Exercise

Continue to spend 10 to 15 minutes writing your own "The Lord is____" devotional prayer of praise. Remember, you don't need to be eloquent to honor God by this exercise. The goal is to acknowledge who He has been, is, and will continue to be in your life. Don't get caught up in making it perfect. It's the pouring out of your heart that brings Him glory.

Week 10 Day 6 | *The Lord Is: A Warrior*

When I think about the Lord, I think of Him in several lights: provider, gracious, father, loving, patient, creator, compassionate, and giver, to name a few. Rarely, if ever, do I think of Him as a warrior. However, when I stop to think about what a warrior does and stands for, it's a perfect description.

First of all, a warrior is someone who fights in battles. We certainly know this is the case with the Lord. He has been involved in battles since He first cast Satan out of heaven. We see throughout the Old Testament where He intervened to give victory to His people.

Moses was certainly no stranger to God's hand in war. Moses witnessed it over the Amalekites, Canaanites, Amorites, and Midianites. Perhaps the most dramatic display of the Lord's warrior nature was at the parting of the Red Sea. God held back walls of water for the Israelites so they could pass, only to let the water crash on the Egyptian army of Pharaoh, Egyptians drowning en masse as their bodies washed up on the shore. After the crossing, Moses first gave the Lord this descriptive title in "The Song of Deliverance":

"The Lord is a warrior; Yahweh is his name!" –Exodus 15:3 (NLT)

Gideon, Joshua, Jephthah, Samuel, Saul, David, and many others were also led by the Lord into battles. In each of them, He—the Warrior—gave them victory.

Secondly, a warrior is someone who is courageous. Now, "courageous" might seem like a strange adjective to ascribe to the God of creation. After all, whom does He have to fear? However, God was courageous to create man, knowing man would turn away. It took courage to keep showing grace and compassion when man kept rejecting Him. It took courage to offer His Son as a sacrifice, knowing His perfect Jesus would take on the weight of the world's sin. It took courage to offer a humanity that rejected God an opportunity to have an eternal life with Him. God has the moral strength to persevere in the face of difficulty. That's courage. That's a warrior.

Warriors secure victory. By their efforts and contributions, their hand in the outcome is undeniable. Without them, success would not be possible. This is something Jeremiah understood fully. The victories he had were only because of his God. He knew the source for his success:

> *"But the Lord stands beside me like a great warrior. Before him my persecutors will stumble. They cannot defeat me."*
> —Jeremiah 20:11 (NLT)

By sacrifice, determination, will, and drive, warriors give everything they have so that victory can be won. Whether they live or die, they will do what must be done so that the objective can be achieved. This too exemplifies our Lord. His very Son died to conquer sin and death, that we would not be eternally defeated, that we could experience true and lasting victory.

We can experience victory with our fitness, too, when we approach it like a warrior prepares for combat. First, we adopt a battle stance, a mindset that this won't be easy. Yet we are willing to fight, to do whatever it takes, no matter what.

Our fitness requires courage . . . a lot of courage. It's hard engaging in a war we've lost so many times before. Getting healthy is difficult knowing the sacrifices we are preparing to make. You have to be brave to battle what might be lifelong demons that attack your self-worth and value. By now, perhaps your nerves are frayed and insecurities are solidified. Yet taking action in spite of this, in spite of all these fears, that is what our courage is all about!

Lastly, fitness requires thinking in terms of victory. True warriors enter battle thinking they will do whatever it takes to win. There is one and only one objective and that's to attain victory at all costs. Our focus is not on "what if" but on the "I will." I will win. I will succeed. I will conquer.

The reason "I will" conquer is because "He does" the conquering. We have the ultimate Victor already on our side. He is commanding the army and empowering it. He is in us, He is at work, and He is leading the charge.

Describing the Lord as a warrior is perfectly fitting. He pursues our hearts with wild abandon. He wins the wars at all costs. Without hesitation, He courageously orchestrates victories on our behalf.

You should be emboldened whenever you're facing your fitness fiends. Food, lethargy, anxieties, previous defeat, or future dread may be at your heels. If so, take a note from Jeremiah and remind yourself of this simple truth: the Warrior of the world stands beside you. The schemes and attacks from the enemy will fail before Him. They cannot defeat you!

While your fitness is a fight, the Lord is the ultimate fighter. He has an undefeated record. Put Him at the head of the attack, follow Him in battle, and see what He has planned. I can't guarantee you'll reach your physical goals, but I can promise He will work your fitness for your good . . . and for the Warrior's glory.

Prayer
Father, thank You for being, among so many other things, a warrior. Will You forgive me when I take for granted how You have battled for my heart? Please help me to live a life characterized by courage rooted in who You are and what You've done. Amen.

Meditation
The Lord is my Warrior.

Daily Spiritual Exercise
Continue to spend 10 to 15 minutes writing your own "The Lord is____" devotional prayer of praise. Remember, you don't need to be eloquent to honor God by this exercise. The goal is to acknowledge who He has been, is, and will continue to be in your life. Don't get caught up in making it perfect. It's the pouring out of your heart that brings Him glory.

Week 10 Day 7 | *The Lord Is: My Refuge*

Have you ever seen the Running of the Bulls? The most famous one is held in Pamplona, Spain. Thousands of adventurers try to outmaneuver, outrun, or outlast a group of bulls released in some blocked-off streets spanning a half-mile. It's an interesting sight to watch people literally run for their lives.

Maybe you've seen a movie where the heroes are being chased as they run for the gates of their country's embassy. Imagine a young boy running home as he is being chased by a pack of bullies. Whatever the case, once they reach their destination, a wave of relief washes over them. They're safe . . . secure . . . protected. They have found refuge.

In Old Testament times, the word "refuge" was especially significant as there were entire cities designated as "Cities of Refuge." Revenge was so prominent that manslaughter was repaid with manslaughter, oftentimes done by the hands of the victim's family, even if the death was unintentional. If you were involved in an accidental death, you could flee to one of six Cities of Refuge. There you were kept safe as you awaited trial. You can imagine an enormous sense of relief washing over you once inside those city walls.

Although King David never fled to a City of Refuge, he certainly knew what it was like to be pursued by his enemies. David's faith, obedience, and love of the Lord's law made him a man after God's own heart (1 Samuel 13:14). As admirable as these traits were, David was more impressive for something else: his complete and utter desperation for the Lord. This is why he was especially fond of referring to the Lord as a "refuge." For David, the Lord as a refuge meant God was a place of safety for the distressed (Psalm 59:16). The Lord was a strong tower that no enemy could breach (Psalm 61:3). He was a shelter that no evil could conquer (Psalm 91:9–10), and under which David could live free of condemnation (Psalm 34:22). The Lord wasn't just "a" refuge for David; He was "the" refuge (Psalm 91:2).

In one of the most revealing, honest declarations of them all, David wrote:

"Then I pray to you, O Lord. I say, 'You are my place of refuge.
You are all I really want in life.'"—Psalm 142:5 (NLT)

Imagine, a king with the world at his fingertips, and all He really wants is the God who is at his side: "You are all I really want in life." All that matters, all that counts, all that's worth anything worth having is the Lord and the safety He provides.

With only three weeks remaining in our fitness journey, you are entering the flare phase. This is when things typically start getting easier and more realistic. The idea that fitness is sustainable is starting to resonate with you.

However, that's not always the case for the flare phase. You may still be feeling that the enemy is in hot pursuit. He's nipping at your heels with reminders of recent failures or setbacks. Your resolve is fading, though the pace of his chasing isn't. To make matters worse, you find yourself believing the growing whispers of defeat you're hearing behind you. You need a City of Refuge.

Provisions were made to ensure accessibility to Cities of Refuge. They were available to everyone, no matter what. The cities were easy to see because they were often built on mountains. The roads leading to the cities were extra wide, well maintained, and never congested. They had plenty of signs and directions posted along the way. Since the gates never closed, once you were there, you were in. If you ever needed a City of Refuge, not only could you get to one, but the city wanted you there.

Sound familiar? It should, because that's the Lord we serve—open to everyone, all the time, no matter what. He's inviting you, welcoming you in, and protecting you once you're there. When we need our City of Refuge—and we need Him every day—we continue running. We know He is strong and good, and will always remain close (Nahum 1:7). We don't stop until we reach our Tower. There, we have shelter from the storms and have shade from the heat (Isaiah 25:4). We put one foot in front of another, knowing He is the One who saves and delivers (Psalm 7:1).

The Lord provides safety and shelter. We should seek to rest in His provision in all circumstances.

Once we arrive, relief washes over us. We're safe . . . secure . . . protected. We have found Refuge. He is all we really need in life.

Prayer

Father, thank You for the safety You provide for us. Will You forgive me when I seek refuge in things that can't provide it? Please help me run to You, all the time, no matter what. Amen.

Meditation

You are my refuge. That is all I need.

Daily Spiritual Exercise

Continue to spend 10 to 15 minutes writing your own "The Lord is____" devotional prayer of praise. Remember, you don't need to be eloquent to honor God by this exercise. The goal is to acknowledge who He has been, is, and will continue to be in your life. Don't get caught up in making it perfect. It's the pouring out of your heart that brings Him glory.

New Testament Heroes

Compared to those in the Old Testament, New Testament heroes feel a little more "blue collar." No kings of nations. No leaders of chosen people. No government dignitaries worth speaking of. Instead, we have fishermen and tax collectors. Carpenters and stay-at-home moms. More "salt of the earth"-type people.

This might explain why the men and women from the New Testament feel more accessible. It's hard to relate to the wisest man who ever lived or a guy who lived inside a fish. Someone who works with his hands for a living? I can identify with someone like that.

New Testament heroes are no less flawed than the Old Testament ones. In some ways, you could argue that they are more so. They had done life with Christ and still had their struggles. They performed miracles with Him and yet denied Him. They had been taught from the Master, yet still could not master the flesh.

Just as with our Old Testament heroes, we can find encouragement in the New Testament heroes, warts and all. This time it's a little different. This time . . . there's Jesus. This time we see firsthand how God in flesh dealt with sinful man. This time, we see how Jesus inspired His followers to live for the One who lived in constant communion with His Father. This time, we have emboldened examples of lives lived post-Resurrection.

At the end of the day, New Testament heroes were like you and me. They were ordinary people that God used in extraordinary ways. He can and will do the same with us if we are open to His leading, like these heroes were.

This week, if your results have plateaued, if your enthusiasm has waned, or your resolve has diminished, take heart. Our New Testament heroes set a great example for us. They experienced eventual victory in the face of loss, setbacks, and uncertainty.

Because there's Jesus . . . you can be victorious too!

Daily Spiritual Exercise: Fast and pray.

Our King is, among other things, unrelenting in the pursuit of our hearts. We want to be the same toward Him. One way to do that is by staying in constant prayer with our Father.

Fasting is a great way to remind us of this need. So, fast from one meal every day. It doesn't matter which meal you choose. Then, whenever you feel hunger pangs, use them as a reminder to be fully surrendered to Him. Pray with thanksgiving for the health He has given you. Pray also that by His Spirit in you, you'd be unrelenting in pursuing your fitness. Most importantly, pray to be unrelenting in pursuing His heart.

Week 11 Day 1 | *New Testament Heroes: Joseph*

Joseph is the Job of the New Testament, in the sense that he gets little of the attention he deserves. At center stage we have the wonders of Mary's virgin birth. Or the mystery of a star leading the Magi. Or the excitement of angels appearing to shepherds. Joseph consistently gets overshadowed in the story of Jesus arrival. Yet Joseph is the essence of a servant of God. He's fully obedient and honorable, a consistent example for anyone called to be faithful in an uncertain time.

We don't know much about Joseph, really. He was a carpenter, the son of Jacob, and a descendant in the line of David. That's about it. What we lack in background details, however, we more than make up for with examples of strong character. Joseph is described as "righteous." The Amplified Bible uses the adjectives "just" and "upright." The New Living Translation describes him as "a good man." We see this on display immediately upon meeting Joseph. We're told that he plans to divorce a pregnant Mary in private, rather than shame her in the open. Keep in mind, he could have demanded her death, as allowed by Old Testament law:

> *"And Joseph her husband, being a righteous man, and not willing to make her a public example, was minded to put her away privily."*
> *—Matthew 1:19 (ASV)*

Not sure about you, but I like him already.

Soon after that, an angel of the Lord appeared to Joseph in a dream. The angel told him to take Mary as his wife and to name the baby Jesus. Matthew 1:24 says, "When Joseph woke up, he did what the angel of the Lord had commanded him and took Mary home as his wife."

You may be thinking, "Yeah, well, if an angel appeared to me, I'd do what it said too." Remember, though, the angel appeared to Joseph in a dream. It would be quite reasonable to question yourself and the validity of what went on in your sleep. Even if the impression was so strong that it couldn't be denied, the Bible is littered with stories of disobedience, not just from an angel's instructions, but from God Himself: Adam, Moses, Samson, and Jonah, to name a few. Not Joseph. There's no evidence of him faltering. No questioning the legitimacy of the virgin birth. No resentment for receiving this unrequested role as a stepfather.

We see this over and over again with Joseph. Escaping from Egypt, in Matthew 2, was an instruction from an angel of the Lord. Returning to Nazareth later in chapter 2, also an instruction from the Lord. In Luke 2, Joseph presented Jesus to the Lord at the Jerusalem temple, where Simeon anointed the infant King. This is Joseph's obedience to the Law of Moses. Then, later in Luke, we see Joseph's faithfulness to return annually to Jerusalem for the Passover.

Just plain . . . old . . . simple . . . obedience. One day at a time. One foot in front of the other. Consistency.

As with Joseph (and Job), consistency is underrated. It doesn't get the spotlight. Frankly, it sounds a little boring.

Spontaneity, now that's fun, right? New. Exciting. Different.

There is great power in consistency. In fact, without it, nothing can change. You can't get stronger in your workouts. You can't improve your race times. You can't progress in your efforts to drop some weight. You can't wake up renewed day after day. You just can't establish a healthy lifestyle without consistency. It doesn't stop with your fitness . . . you can't become a better parent or child or sibling without it. You can't become a better friend, employee, or citizen without it.

With consistency, good things can happen. With consistent obedience, amazing things happen. There is growth! Change is realized. Goals are achieved. Potential is reached. With consistency, your walk with Christ becomes the most exciting, fulfilling, purposeful, triumphant journey your life will ever know.

Stop trying to be clever in your walk with God. Don't look for fancy ways to bring God glory if you're not glorifying Him in the simplest of ways. Consistent obedience in matters great and small may not sound profound, but the results of it are. Just ask Joseph.

Prayer

Father, thank You for Your consistent availability. Will You forgive me when I don't consistently rely on the indwelling of the Holy Spirit? Please change me. Help me to trust You to accomplish Your purposes through me, just as Joseph did. Amen.

Meditation

To be consistently obedient, I will consistently rely on You.

Daily Spiritual Exercise

Pick a meal to fast from for the day. The hunger you feel is a reminder to be praying for a fully surrendered life. As you pray throughout the day, be sure to ask God what He'd like you to learn from this exercise. We don't just pray. We pray and we listen.

Week 11 Day 2 | *New Testament Heroes: The Centurion*

We are amazed by Jesus, but perhaps not amazed often enough. He taught in the synagogues and healed the sick (Matthew 4:23). He cast out demons and raised the dead (Mark 5). He forgave sins (Matthew 5:20) and conquered death (Luke 24). The Gospel of John tells us that there aren't enough books in the world that could contain all that Jesus did (John 21:25).

Jesus was nothing short of amazing. When someone that incredible is said to have been "amazed" Himself, we should stop and take notice. One such time was in regard to today's New Testament hero, the centurion.

Matthew 8 or Luke 7 both tell the story of the centurion. Read either and you'll find at least three things that stand out about this man: his love, humility, and faith. Any one of those attributes can stand alone as a source of encouragement to us. Stack one on top of the other, however, and it's easy to see why Jesus was amazed by the centurion.

If you're unfamiliar with the story, a centurion was concerned over his dying servant. The centurion sent some respected friends to Jesus so Jesus could heal this servant. Jesus agreed to come but was stopped before entering the house. The centurion did not feel worthy to have Jesus in his house. On behalf of the centurion, his friends asked Jesus to "say the word," knowing those words would be sufficient for healing of the centurion's servant. We then read that Jesus "was amazed." When the centurion's friends had returned to his house, they found the servant healed.

Having some background will make this story all the more inspiring. A centurion was a commander of 100 soldiers in the Roman army. A man of his authority could very well have had many servants. Furthermore, it wouldn't have been uncommon to treat them poorly. Not this centurion. Luke 7:2 tells us He "valued highly" his servant. The centurion cared so much that he sent for help from Jesus for the man who was "paralyzed, suffering terribly." The centurion showed great love where none would have been expected.

Then, when Jesus graciously asks if He should come and heal the servant, we see the centurion's great humility emerge. Luke 7:6–7 recounts the story: "Lord, don't trouble yourself, for I do not deserve to have you come under my roof. That is why I did not even consider myself worthy to come to you." In spite of the centurion's earthly position, of his vast resources, and of being well respected (Luke 7:4–5), he remained humble. The centurion understood that these meant very little compared to the One who had been given all authority in heaven and earth. The centurion's heart was greater than his status.

Next, we see the centurion's great faith. Luke 7:7 continues, "But say the word, and my servant will be healed." It's faith enough to believe that Jesus could touch the servant and the servant would be healed. Yet to believe that words alone would be sufficient displays a deepness of trust rarely seen in Scripture:

> "When Jesus heard this, he was amazed and said to those following him, 'Truly I tell you, I have not found anyone in Israel with such great faith.'"–Matthew 8:10 (NIV)

The centurion's faith in Jesus' power was affirmed. Matthew 8:13 concludes the story this way: "Then Jesus said to the centurion, 'Go! Let it be done just as you believed it would.' And his servant was healed at that moment."

Love. Humility. Faith. I think it's fair to say these traits characterized the centurion. Here's what's exciting: such attributes can characterize us too. We are already blessed because we believe but have not seen (John 20:29). The Holy Spirit lives in us (1 Corinthians 3:16). We have access to the One who marked the heavens with the breadth of His hands (Isaiah 40:12). Therefore, Jesus being "amazed" doesn't have to be confined only to the story of the centurion.

When a woman forgives a drunk driver for killing her husband, God is amazed. When an 82-year-old repents for his hardened life of rebellion and indulgence, God is amazed. When a family praises the Father in spite of cancer stealing their mom, God is amazed. When the lone Christian stands up for her faith in the face of her atheist professor, God is amazed. When the stay-at-home mom turns from food to God for her ultimate source of comfort, God is amazed.

He is amazed . . . but not surprised.

If we want to amaze God and be amazed by God, love others, stay humble, and keep your faith first.

We can all be centurions.

Prayer

Father, thank You for marveling at anything I might do. Will You forgive me when I fail to be amazed by You? By your Spirit in me, make me more like the centurion. Grow my love. Establish my humility. Increase my faith. Amen.

Meditation

Work in me that my love, faith and humility might amaze for your kingdom.

Daily Spiritual Exercise

Pick a meal to fast from for the day. The hunger you feel is a reminder to be praying for a fully surrendered life. As you pray throughout the day, be sure to ask God what He'd like you to learn from this exercise. We don't just pray. We pray and we listen.

Week 11 Day 3 – *New Testament Heroes: The Widow*

In Gary Chapman's excellent book *The Five Love Languages*, he categorizes what he believes are the five primary expressions of love: acts of service, encouraging words, quality time, physical touch, and gift giving. Generally, you have one or two of these love languages that take precedence in how you love and how you feel loved. This is extraordinarily helpful when cultivating relationships with your friends and family. My primary love language is gift giving.

This goes back to my youth, though I didn't realize it at the time. I can recall one December in particular when I was in middle school. The most wonderful time of the year was upon us. I remember spending hours at the mall shopping for my friends. I was searching for the perfect gift for each one of them. Using my own hard-earned money, I selected a stuffed animal for Jenny that I thought she would love. An awesome action figure for Johnny. The perfect game for Billy, and so on. I must have spent close to $75, which in the mid-'80s was a lot of money for a 12-year-old.

The day of the great gift exchange came and, unfortunately, it did not go well for me. Let's just say, my friends and I didn't share the same love language. I got the royal shaft (if I got anything at all), and I was devastated. Now in fairness to my friends, it wasn't as if they didn't love me, nor was it necessarily how they expressed their friendship. What was so hard for me were my expectations. I gave my all and got very little in return.

Has this ever happened to you? Have you ever given your all to something and then have nothing to show for it? More specifically, have you given your fitness your all and then didn't get anything back? The scale didn't move. No new PR (personal record) in a race. You're not lifting heavier weights, seeing your cholesterol or blood pressure go down, or recovery time improve? It's really hard, right? It's discouraging. Makes you want to give up. Not getting results . . . then why bother?

In a situation like this, you can adopt one of two attitudes. I've coached people through them both. Each choice leads to different outcomes. The first attitude can be found in the story of the rich young ruler depicted in all four of the Gospels.

The wealthy young ruler went to Jesus and asked what he should do to earn eternal life for himself. When Jesus told the man to sell everything and follow Him, the ruler felt great sorrow because he was rich. In other words, the cost was too high. The young man was comfortable where he was. The required sacrifice was too great, or the reward was too small, or both. The man's heart was only focused on himself and on the present.

When people have a selfish, nearsighted attitude toward their fitness, it eventually breaks them. They quit because they don't see results. Or, if they do start seeing results, that becomes their focus rather than God. Quitting or having a misaligned focus is at best a missed opportunity to bring God glory. At worst, it's a slippery slope to idolatry.

On the flipside, we can have the attitude of the poor widow mentioned in Scripture:

> *"As Jesus looked up, he saw the rich putting their gifts into the temple treasury. He also saw a poor widow put in two very small copper coins. 'Truly I tell you,' he said, 'this poor widow has put in more than all the others. All these people gave their gifts out of their wealth; but she out of her poverty put in all she had to live on.'"*
> *—Luke 21:1–4 (NIV)*

Even though it didn't amount to much, the widow gave all she had. No matter how it affected her and with indifference to how much it actually contributed to the offering, she gave.

That's how you can reorient your fitness in a God-glorifying away. Adopt that same mindset of giving your all, without regard to how it affects you and indifferent to the results you achieve. Then, your fitness not only becomes easier, it becomes more enjoyable.

I've seen many people struggle with various legitimate health issues, sometimes battling multiple complications at the same time. They don't usually see the results they're wanting. Yet they still find joy in their fitness because their hearts are aligned with His heart, not with their results.

This joy and dedication pleases our Lord because out of the poverty of their health, they are giving Him all they have.

Remember my Great Christmas Debacle of '86? How much more would I have enjoyed the fun of giving if I had no expectations for the outcome? I could have simply absorbed the smiles of my friends as they opened their presents. I could have laughed with them as they played with their games. My heart would have been aligned with the Giver of every good gift. I could have found joy strictly in the process of giving because I would have not been focused on myself.

That's why when it comes to our fitness, we first concern ourselves with the heart. Joyfully giving out of our poverty, we present our fitness as an offering. We should expect nothing but trust God with everything.

When we pursue our fitness with a clean heart, no matter how poor our results, we will be rich in Him. That's the best result of all.

Prayer
Father, thank You for accepting my fitness as an offering of love to You. Will You forgive me when I'm motivated for and by the wrong things? Help me to give You my all no matter what. Amen.

Meditation
Give me a clean heart, keeping you the focus of my fitness.

Daily Spiritual Exercise
Pick a meal to fast from for the day. The hunger you feel is a reminder to be praying for a fully surrendered life. As you pray throughout the day, be sure to ask God what He'd like you to learn from this exercise. We don't just pray. We pray and we listen.

Week 11 Day 4 | *New Testament Heroes: Zacchaeus*

The story of Zacchaeus is one of the more famous stories in the Bible, thanks in part to the children's song. If you're unfamiliar with this classic Sunday school staple, it goes like this:

> *Zacchaeus was a wee little man*
> *and a wee little man was he.*
> *He climbed up in a sycamore tree*
> *for the Lord he wanted to see.*
>
> *And as the Savior passed that way*
> *He looked up in that tree.*
> *And He said, "Zacchaeus, you come down!*
> *For I'm going to your house today!*
> *For I'm going to your house today!"*

We can learn a lot from this little guy, especially what is left out of the song.

Zacchaeus was a tax collector. Well, people didn't like tax collectors due to the very nature of their job. Many tax collectors abused their position as a way to increase their personal wealth. They mercilessly overcharged their neighbors, keeping the excess for themselves. So when Luke 19:2 states that Zacchaeus was a "chief" tax collector and was rich, it's fair to assume he took advantage of his position. If people didn't like Zacchaeus, who could blame them?

For some reason, though, Zacchaeus wanted to know more about Jesus. In verse 3, we read, "And he was seeking to see who Jesus was...." Certainly, Jesus drew a crowd and perhaps Zacchaeus was merely curious. However, based on Zacchaeus' response to Jesus later on, my guess is that God was stirring in Zacchaeus' heart. Perhaps this was God planting the seeds of true life change.

Similarly, God might be doing the same with your heart even now. You sense His moving in your life, though you're unsure how or why or with what exactly. The question then becomes, how are you going to respond?

Let's look at how Zacchaeus responded. Luke 19:4 tells us that before he climbed the tree, "… he ran ahead…." Zacchaeus was determined! Neither the height, nor the size, nor the pace of the crowd was going to stop Zacchaeus from seeing Jesus. He ran and scurried up that tree to catch a glimpse of Jesus.

We should ask ourselves: do we truly seek Jesus with determination? Will we stop at nothing to see Him, know Him, and learn more about Him? Are we striving to see what He can do in our lives, including our fitness lives?

After Zacchaeus perched himself in the tree, we read in verse 5 that Jesus said, "Zacchaeus, hurry and come down, for I must stay at your house today."

Zacchaeus' response is stellar:

> *"So he hurried and came down and received him joyfully."*
> *—verse 6 (ESV)*

Jesus tells Zacchaeus to hurry and Zacchaeus hurries. Complete obedience. Not only does he obey completely, He does so joyfully.

How do you respond when you "hear" from God, in Scripture, through friends, convictions from the Holy Spirit, at church, in a book, or wherever? Once you know what you're supposed to do, how do you respond? When He tells you to "hurry," do you take your time? We might already know what God would have us do, including where our fitness is concerned. Yet we only respond partially and begrudgingly. Rather than committing to clean eating with a grateful heart, we reluctantly eat an occasional salad. Instead of faithfully and joyfully pursuing exercise, we consider retail therapy at the mall to be our workout for the day.

This is not how Zacchaeus would have embraced his fitness. He would have passionately, earnestly, and joyfully pursued God-honoring body stewardship. Little Zacchaeus sets a big-time example.

In verse 7, we see the crowd's reaction: "And when they saw it, they all grumbled, 'He has gone in to be the guest of a man who is a sinner.'"

People didn't like Zacchaeus and they didn't like that Jesus wanted to spend time with Zacchaeus. However, that didn't matter to Zacchaeus . . . or to Jesus.

Many people won't like it when you want to make a life change with your fitness either. This may be especially true when you want to include Jesus in the process. That shouldn't matter to you, because it doesn't matter to Jesus. Besides, you never know . . . the excitement rekindling here in Week 11 of this journey could speak to others. God could use your example to convict them or as a catalyst for them to get started with their fitness. Or better yet, God could use you to get them to seek Jesus in all areas of their life, including their fitness.

Moving on to Luke 19:8, we see a changed man: "And Zacchaeus stood and said to the Lord, 'Behold, Lord, the half of my goods I give to the poor. And if I have defrauded anyone of anything, I restore it fourfold.'" Zacchaeus, the disliked, tax-collecting sinner, went all-in.

As Jesus goes on to tell us in Luke 19:9, salvation had come to this house!

Let's recap: We need to seek Jesus with determination. When He talks, we should respond completely and joyfully. We don't concern ourselves with what the world thinks because we don't live for the world. When we commit, we do so authentically.

Our response to God's calling should be fervent, complete, and joyful. The same should be said about our fitness. We are not honoring God if we're grumbling and half-hearted in our efforts. As always, honoring God with our bodies begins by honoring Him with our hearts.

So take a cue from Zacchaeus. Be passionate, earnest and joyful in your pursuit of the Lord . . . knowing you will be going to His house someday.

Prayer

Father, thank You for getting me this far, not just in my fitness, but in my life. Will You forgive me when I don't obey You fully, fervently, and joyfully? Help me always stay determined, faithful, and authentic in my walk with You. Amen.

Meditation

I will seek You passionately, joyfully, and completely.

Daily Spiritual Exercise

Pick a meal to fast from for the day. The hunger you feel is a reminder to be praying for a fully surrendered life. As you pray throughout the day, be sure to ask God what He'd like you to learn from this exercise. We don't just pray. We pray and we listen.

Week 11 Day 5 | *New Testament Heroes: The Sick Woman*

How would you complete this sentence? If I just_____, then _____.

Perhaps you'd say, "If I just got that raise, then we could pay our bills." "If I just got married, then I'd be happy." "If I just quit my job, then life would be better." "If I just lost 30 pounds, then I'd look pretty." "If I just got a little stronger. A little faster. Had more discipline. Got more sleep . . . then I'd be healthier."

The truth is, there's always more to want in this world, but none of it satisfies for long. No worldly achievement. No relationship. No amount of money. No job. No result in the mirror, on the scale, in the gym, or on the racecourse. Because no sooner do you reach one of these goals than you change your answer. You will fill in the blank with something else. However, in the New Testament, we read about a woman who filled in the blank perfectly the first time.

Mark 5 recounts three of the many miracles Jesus performed, each indelible in its own way. We first read about Jesus healing Legion, a man possessed with thousands of demons. The last one we read about is a young girl being resurrected. It's the one in the middle, the story of the sick woman, that we can relate to most easily.

The story begins in verse 25: "And a woman was there who had been subject to bleeding for twelve years." That's a long time to be sick. It's a long time to be suffering. Do you, too, have a long-standing ailment of some kind? Could it be a different kind of suffering: addiction, relational, or occupational? Have you struggled with being over- or under-weight, eating disorders, or an unhealthy self-esteem—be it pride or negative self-worth? Whatever it is, we, like the sick woman, have all gone through legitimate sufferings in our lives, some lasting many, many years.

Mark 5:26a continues, "She had suffered a great deal under the care of many doctors and had spent all she had . . ." She had sought professional help, but no one was able to help her. In fact, she had seen so many doctors that she had used up all her money. Sound familiar?

Perhaps you've seen doctors or counselors, and read all the latest self-help books. You've attended workshops, listened to podcasts and sermons, and subscribed to medical journals. You've tried the latest fad diets, done all the Hollywood exercise plans. You've both ignored fitness and been consumed by it. In the process, you've spent a small fortune. That's the story of this sick woman.

Verse 26b finishes, ". . . yet instead of getting better she grew worse." To add insult to injury, not only didn't she get healthier, she got sicker. She had nothing to show for her efforts. Her health was going and her wealth was gone.

Starting to relate? Could it be that you are worse off now than when you started? Your weight is at an all-time high or a life-threatening low. Your race times are getting longer. Your sleep is getting shorter. Your fatigue is going up while your confidence is going down. You're more frustrated, confused, obsessed, and hopeless than ever.

The sick woman was also hopeless until . . . until she remembered Jesus. There were large crowds wherever He went. He had just freed a man from demon possession and was on His way to free a girl from death. Jesus was in this poor lady's midst and this was her chance. Her story continues:

> "When she heard about Jesus, she came up behind him in the crowd and touched his cloak, because she thought, 'If I just touch his clothes, I will be healed.'"–Mark 5:27 (NIV)

The woman was healed immediately. Jesus tells her in verse 34, "Daughter, your faith has healed you. Go in peace and be freed from your suffering."

You see, no longer was her cure about seeing the so-called experts. Her treatment would not require spending money. Healing certainly was not coming from her own efforts. The remedy wasn't about anything this world had to offer anymore. The solution was Jesus. The medicine is Jesus.

Although Jesus may or may not cure our suffering, we can have peace and hope in the midst of it. We have the same opportunity as the bleeding woman. We can follow her lead, be broken and desperate, and have faith only in Jesus. No matter what suffering we are facing. No matter what we've tried before. No matter what results we've seen. No matter our past, present, or future. He promises that we will not be disappointed in our hope (Romans 5:5).

So, now, let me ask again. How would you complete this sentence? If I just_____, then_____.

Are you tired of getting your hopes up and then letting yourself down? Are you exhausted from fear, despair, and disappointment? If in Week 11 you're worse off than you were in Week 1, it's time to change your answer.

If you are not seeing results in your fitness, are you reaching for Jesus first? If you are reaching, do you truly believe in His power to help you? Don't go through the motions with your fitness or your faith!

Take a cue from the sick woman with the perfect answer: "If I just touch Jesus."

When you do, don't let go. Trust Him with the results, because in the end, He is the only One who truly heals.

Prayer
Father, thank You that amid a temporary world, we have an everlasting love in You. Will You forgive me when I base my satisfaction on things that can't satisfy? Please help me to reach only for your Son, Jesus. Amen.

Meditation
I'm healed by the touch of Jesus.

Daily Spiritual Exercise
Pick a meal to fast from for the day. The hunger you feel is a reminder to be praying for a fully surrendered life. As you pray throughout the day, be sure to ask God what He'd like you to learn from this exercise. We don't just pray. We pray and we listen.

Week 11 Day 6 | *New Testament Heroes: Mary*

Like Joseph, Mary's response to the news of the birth of Jesus offers many lessons about living a life characterized by faith and obedience.

We all know the general story of Jesus' birth. Gabriel, an angel of the Lord, appears to Mary, a virgin engaged to be married. The angel reveals that Mary would give birth to the Son of God. Nine-ish months later, Joseph and Mary travel to Bethlehem, where Jesus is born. Shepherds see some angels and rush off to see the Messiah lying in a manger.

It's easy to overlook some rather important details that make Mary's response to the situation so extraordinary, such as her age. Mary was likely only 12 or 13 when Gabriel informed her of the news that she was pregnant.

Also extraordinary was Gabriel. His appearing to Mary was a miracle in and of itself, and miracles weren't all that common. Witnessing something that happened so seldomly would be a spectacle at any age, let alone to someone so young.

Then factor in that the miracle itself: Mary, a virgin, will be giving birth to the Son of God and He will change the course of human history. Talk about pressure!

Upon hearing all this, we read Mary's simple reply:

> *"Mary responded, 'I am the Lord's servant. May everything you have said about me come true.'"*—Luke 1:38 (NLT)

She didn't say, "Why me? Can't someone else do it?" She didn't reply, "I'm not ready for kids. I really just want to get married and have some 'me and Joseph time,' because, you know, once you're a parent, you're always a parent."

We see no indication that Mary was concerned about the looks she would get, being an unwed, pregnant teen. Think the stigma is rough now? Back then, it would have looked like adultery, which was punishable by death by stoning. Yet, Mary shows a willing and fearless obedience with five simple words: "I am the Lord's servant."

After Gabriel appeared to Mary, we read that Mary went to see her cousin Elizabeth, who has experienced a miracle of her own (Luke 1:5–25). Upon hearing Mary's greeting, Elizabeth is filled with the Holy Spirit. In Luke 1:45 Elizabeth says, "You are blessed because you believed that the Lord would do what he said." Mary's obedience is reinforced by her faith. For some people, obedience and faith can be mutually exclusive. Not for Mary.

In Luke 1:46–55 we have Mary's response. Scholars call it "The Magnificat." In this song of praise, she details her blessings. Mary also acclaims the great provision and mercy that God the Savior has for His people. In the song, she refers to herself as "his lowly servant girl" (verse 48). By referring to "his," she establishes to whom she belongs. Then by describing herself as "lowly servant girl," she acknowledges her role in His plan. Once again, just like in her response to Gabriel, Mary's response reinforces her mature humility.

Mary understands the source of her true wealth and hope. We're told in Luke 2:19, "but Mary kept all these things in her heart and thought about them often." She made a habit of counting her blessings and remembering the significance of Jesus' arrival. In addition to her humility, Mary displayed ongoing gratitude and kept an intentional awareness of what God was doing.

Now think back to the sort of things you were into when you were Mary's age. Can you recall how mature you were when you were 12 or 13? What would you have done if an angel of God appeared to you? How would you have reacted to the idea of being a parent at that age? How would you have handled being told you would usher in the Savior of all mankind?

I didn't like waking up on Saturdays to a list of chores to do before I could play Nintendo. Tell me my childhood was over, I was going to be a parent, my son was to be called Jesus, Jesus was also the Son of God, and His kingdom would never end? My first thought would probably be, "I don't even get to name him?" I certainly would not have responded like Mary did.

We aren't often asked to obey in events that are going to change the history of the world. We are asked to obey God in the "everyday" events, including those involving body stewardship. What if we modeled our approach to fitness after Mary's response to Gabriel and ultimately to God? We know in our heart that we need to exercise, eat, and sleep better as a way of life. Yet we're reluctant. Instead, what if we just responded with simple obedience?

What if we stopped fearfully questioning whether our efforts were do-able, sustainable, or productive? What if, instead, we had faith that God would work out what He willed in the first place?

Rather than counting the cost, what if we consistently considered the blessing of His provision in our lives instead? What if we were humble and ever-thankful to the Lord? What if we simply trusted that what He requires of us, He will provide for us?

What if . . . from this point forward . . . you responded to your fitness with "I am the Lord's servant?" What if you responded to your entire life that way? How much more abundant, productive, and fulfilling of a life could the Lord live through you?

Now, before you start thinking you couldn't do that, let me share five other words even more powerful than Mary's. They actually preceded Mary's in "The Magnificat," and gave her full confidence to respond with complete submissiveness. In fact, their truth precedes the creation of the world. They manifest themselves daily in the glue holding life together. They pave the way for a life lived in perfect eternity:

> *". . . nothing is impossible with God."–Luke 1:37 (NLT)*

If these five words can change the world, could they not also change your life as they did for Mary?

Mary responded as a servant. We, too, would be wise to adopt a servants' mindset with our faith and fitness. We can then trust that the One who came not to be served but to serve will work wonders in our lives.

Prayer

Father, thank You for choosing a young servant girl as a model of humility, faith, and obedience. Will You please forgive me when my life is not characterized by those same qualities? Please help me always rely on You as my strength for everything, knowing it's all possible because of You. Amen.

Meditation

Nothing is impossible with God.

Daily Spiritual Exercise

Pick a meal to fast from for the day. The hunger you feel is a reminder to be praying for a fully surrendered life. As you pray throughout the day, be sure to ask God what He'd like you to learn from this exercise. We don't just pray. We pray and we listen.

Week 11 Day 7 | *New Testament Heroes: Silas*

Silas, like Joseph and Job, is another unsung hero in the Bible. People such as Moses, David, John the Baptist, Peter, and Paul seem to get all the glory, while lesser-mentioned greats like Silas fly under the radar. Yet their faith is equally impressive. If we study them and give them the attention they deserve, we see that their example can be equally influential.

A Jew with Roman citizenship (and the Roman name of "Silvanus"), Silas is described by Luke as one of the leaders of the believers in the church (Acts 15:22). Silas was also a prophet whose preaching did a great deal to encourage and strengthen the faith of the church (Acts 15:32). If you can count the quality of a man by the company he keeps, Silas was of the highest quality. Not only was he a scribe for Peter, Silas was surrounded by other "prominent" believers (Acts 17:4). However, he's probably most well known for being Paul's partner on his second missionary journey.

This is where Silas starts to feel like Scottie Pippen to Paul's Michael Jordan, or Robin to Paul's Batman. Paul gets the limelight, but Silas is with him nearly every step along the way. Silas preached with Paul in Berea (Acts 17:10) and Corinth (2 Corinthians 1:19). However, it was their time together in Philippi that best reveals Silas' character.

In Acts 16, Silas and Paul were unjustly dragged out into the public square after Paul healed a girl of her demon possession. Once in front of the authorities, they were lied about, stripped, beaten, and thrown into prison. While their feet were clamped in stocks, they sat disgraced and in pain under the watch of a jailer.

What would you do in this situation? Cry? Cuss? Complain? All of the above? I'm not sure what I would've done, but I'm pretty sure it wouldn't have been what Silas and Paul did:

> *"About midnight Paul and Silas were praying and singing hymns to God, and the other prisoners were listening to them."—Acts 16:25 (NIV)*

Say what? You free a girl from an evil spirit, you're chastened, chained and beaten for it, and you respond with worship? You praise Jesus, for whose sake you were thrown in jail in the first place? You point back to Jesus?

You see, Silas and Paul's circumstances didn't *change* their beliefs; they *revealed* them. You don't see Silas blaming Paul: "Look at what you've gotten me into!" They didn't question, challenge, or complain about God's plan. Instead, they trusted that God would stay true to God's character. Lo and behold, in the very next verse, God delivers.

An earthquake shook, prison doors flew open and prison chains fell off. When the jailer saw what had happened, he figured the prisoners had escaped. So, he drew his sword to kill himself, knowing he'd be executed for it anyway. Paul shouted to stop the jailer, as no prisoner had escaped. Then, the trembling jailer asked Silas and Paul what he needed to do to be saved. Once again, Silas and Paul used their circumstances to advance the gospel. They used their situation to point back to Jesus:

> **"Then they spoke the word of the Lord to him and to all the others in his house."—Acts 16:32 (NIV)**

Silas and Paul remained faithful, in spite of their circumstances. God, in His glorious faithfulness, then used them to bring the jailer and his family into His fold (Acts 16:33–34).

Now, just for a second, let's say there was no earthquake—the chains never fell off, the doors never opened, and Silas and Paul died in prison. Would this sully or tarnish God's character? Would the Lord be any less faithful if He had not set Silas and Paul free? Of course not. The goodness of God's character lies not in what He does or allows, but in who He is.

If we confuse the two, it becomes a "what have you done for me lately" relationship . . . loving with conditional love. Silas and Paul knew the difference, even though they did not know the future. They humbly demonstrated their faith through their praying and singing following their incarceration, always pointing back to Jesus.

We, too, would be wise to remain faithful in all things, regardless of our circumstances. "All things" includes our fitness. We want to be praying and praising, whether or not we see results. That way, whether God sends an earthquake or not, we can be found faithful. Whether we break through a new plateau or get hit with another setback, we're assured that we're honoring God with our heart.

Our heart is always our first priority. After that, we can trust God with the rest. What God did with "the rest" of Silas and Paul's time in Philippi didn't end with the jailer:

> *"After Paul and Silas came out of the prison, they went to Lydia's house, where they met with the brothers and sisters and encouraged them. Then they left."—Acts 16:40 (NIV)*

It's just like God to use the situation for one more piece of good. He allowed Silas and Paul to "encourage" the believers, pointing back to Jesus once again.

"Then they left." Just like that, they're gone from Philippi. It kind of fits Silas' personality, if you think about it. There for a moment . . . then gone—quietly weaving his way in and out of the New Testament, maintaining his humility and tenacity and integrity.

Silas was content being used by God however, wherever, and whenever God needed Him, regardless of the outcome. Oh, to have my life characterized in the same light . . . ever pointing back to Jesus.

Are you content with how God is using you for His purposes? Have you considered that He may have a plan for even your fitness, whether it's going strong or not? God used Silas' situations, whether favorable or not, for God's glory. He can do the same for you.

Prayer
Father, thank You for Silas and for his example to remain faithful in all situations. Will You please forgive me when I let my circumstances dictate my response? Please develop in me a heartfelt and steadfast obedience. Amen.

Meditation
I will praise You . . . no matter what.

Daily Spiritual Exercise
Pick a meal to fast from for the day. The hunger you feel is a reminder

to be praying for a fully surrendered life. As you pray throughout the day, be sure to ask God what He'd like you to learn from this exercise. We don't just pray. We pray and we listen.

WEEK 12 PREVIEW

The Fruit of the Spirit

"But the Holy Spirit produces this kind of fruit in our lives: love, joy, peace, patience, kindness, goodness, faithfulness, gentleness, and self-control. There is no law against these things!"—Galatians 5:22–23 (NLT)

It's always a little puzzling, if not troubling, when I hear Christians say, "I don't have that much self-control." "I don't have the patience for that." "I don't think I could ever love so-and-so." Red flags go up because they are not understanding the work of the Holy Spirit.

Living a Spirit-filled life is foremost about what the Holy Spirit does in us and through us. Galatians 5:22 says the Holy Spirit "produces" this kind of fruit in our lives. We don't produce it; He does.

Gardening illustrates the relationship we have with the Holy Spirit. A seed will only grow and produce fruit if certain conditions are met. The soil must be fertile and kept at the right temperature. The seed must receive adequate water and sun. When these requirements are satisfied, fruit is produced. If one or more of these dynamics is out of balance or missing, the harvest is compromised.

Similarly, in order for the Holy Spirit to produce fruit in us, we have to provide the right environment in our heart. To establish fertile grounds, we must start with regular Bible reading, faithful prayer, and Christian fellowship, and include praise and worship. It doesn't stop there, though. We can't just learn to speak "Christianese" and "do churchy things" and expect fruit. That's not the fertile environment the Holy Spirit requires or desires. Providing the right soil also requires relying on and remaining obedient to the Holy Spirit and His leading. When we offer our hearts with this kind of surrendered reliance on the Holy Spirit, He bears fruit . . . in abundance.

This good news is both liberating and exciting! Liberating as it frees us from the burden of producing fruit out of our own efforts. It's exciting because His work is immeasurably more productive, satisfying, and enriching than ours.

If the Holy Spirit is in control, then the fruit is infinite. When the Holy Spirit produces self-control in our lives, for instance, it's coming from a perfect and endless well, one that never runs dry and never leaves us thirsty.

This, too, is liberating and exciting. It's liberating because we are free to enjoy the fruit to the full without fear it will ever be depleted. It's exciting because this same fruit is a testimony to the power of God working in a personal relationship in the lives of His children.

Finally, Christians all have the same Holy Spirit and the same endless supply of the same fruit. One Christian doesn't have "more" of one fruit of the Spirit than another Christian. The Holy Spirit might produce more of one kind of fruit in us, depending on our needs, situations, and prayers. That fruit, however, is not an ability with which we are born. It is God working in us and through us to glorify Himself, not us.

Once again, we should feel liberated and excited. We are liberated from the compulsion to compare ourselves to others or wish we were born different or "better." We should be excited because we can be characterized by love, joy, peace, patience, kindness, goodness, faithfulness, gentleness, and self-control.

When that happens, others see something different in us. They might not know what it is. They just know they want it. They will want the Holy Spirit and the fruit He bears in the lives of Christians.

When the Holy Spirit lives in and through them, they also will be liberated and excited—liberated from the same burdens that weigh us down and excited at the power He provides to lift us up.

The fruit of the Spirit is evidence of the work of the Holy Spirit in your life. When you live a Spirit-filled life, you *can* have the self-control you need. You *can* have the patience others deserve. You *can* exhibit the love God desires. When you are in tune with the Holy Spirit and follow in obedience, there's no limit to what He will do for your life . . . let alone your fitness.

Daily Spiritual Exercise: Focus on a fruit of the Spirit.

Each day this week, pick a different fruit of the Spirit to focus on and celebrate. Remember, these are not "fruits of ourselves." These are the outcomes of the Holy Spirit working in and through our lives.

As you focus on the fruit of the Spirit, pray for wisdom. You may need help in discerning whether you're working out of your efforts and gifts or allowing the Holy Spirit to work.

Hint: The less effort it takes for you to exhibit the fruit of the Spirit, the more it's Him doing the work. If it feels like a total strain, it's probably you relying too much on yourself. When that happens and you're working out of your own strength, use the practice of spiritual breathing you learned in Week 5.

Also, pray for His strength. You'll need it to act on the wisdom He provides, as He nudges your heart in His perfect way.

Week 12 Day 1 | *Fruit of the Spirit: Self-Control*

Ever heard the expression "The best offense is a good defense?" Athletes say it all the time. Take basketball, for example. A team with a quick-handed point guard might be able to steal the ball and score. Taller teams generally block more shots, which can also lead to points. Teams that position themselves better for rebounds can more easily make long passes downcourt for easier baskets.

We see this in football, hockey, soccer, and a host of other sports. In each case, a team's strong defense can lead to points.

"The best offense is a good defense" can be applied to other areas too, like business, politics, and certainly military combat. A strong defense is imperative for victory.

It used to be that cities were literally surrounded by walls, with few ways to enter. These walls were a city's primary defense, especially when actively engaged in war.

For instance, the walls of Jericho were thought to be 5 feet thick and up to 17 feet tall. The walls of Jerusalem were even more impressive, at up to 8 feet thick and nearly 40 feet tall. With walls this tall and thick, the defense had a great advantage when under attack. A city with such a wall had a better vantage point, and the reinforced walls were hard to penetrate, assuming the walls were intact. If the integrity of the wall was compromised with holes or gaps, however, it was a great liability. Suddenly, the city was at a disadvantage because the citizens were boxed in if the enemy invaded.

Take a look at this proverb:

> *"A person without self-control is like a city with broken-down walls."—Proverbs 25:28 (NLT)*

In other words, without self-control, our defense diminishes greatly. We give the enemy openings to climb through, rubble to walk over, and a path to victory.

I like how the Amplified Bible puts that same verse: "He who has no rule over his own spirit is like a city that is broken down and without walls." The problem is we are very poor rulers of ourselves. We let our emotions dictate our actions. Feelings precede facts. Flesh governs over truth.

We'd be far better off if we didn't lead our daily lives. This is where living a Spirit-filled life gets really exciting: we don't have to. In fact, we're not even supposed to! We are not called to be in control of our own spirit. Rather, we are to allow the Holy Spirit to bear the fruit of self-control in us. That's His role, not ours. We can't do it on our own, but He can, He wants to, and He will.

When temptation to skip a workout looms, we rely on the Holy Spirit to bear His fruit of self-control in us. We can then make the right choice. When desire hits to continue making poor choices with our nutrition, we rely on the Holy Spirit. He can stir in us the resolve to choose the healthy options and the right quantities. When we think we'd be better off spending another hour watching TV, we rely on the Holy Spirit. He'll remind us how beneficial sleep is and we can feel empowered to hit the remote and head to bed. The Holy Spirit's nudging to make healthy choices will prevail, if we are willing to listen and follow through in obedience.

The problem of having self-discipline is not usually an awareness issue; it's an obedience issue. When we feel his leading and then follow in obedience, He responds by fortifying our faith and accomplishing His will.

That's the promise of the Holy Spirit at work within us. When He bears the fruit . . . He builds the wall . . . He defends our city.

Prayer
Father, thank You for the fruit of self-control. Will You forgive me when I ignore Your whisper? I know that I cannot do this on my own. I know that You will do this through me, for You. Amen.

Meditation
Self-control is the Holy Spirit's fruit, not mine.

Daily Spiritual Exercise

Today you will focus on the fruit of self-control. Remember, these are not "fruits of ourselves." These are the outcomes of the Holy Spirit working in and through our lives.

As you are focusing on the fruit of self-control, pray for wisdom. You may need help in discerning whether you're working out of your own efforts or allowing the Holy Spirit to work.

Also, be sure to be teachable. Sometimes we are being taught a lesson we don't want to learn. If we are truly open to the Lord working in our lives, however, we need to humbly receive all He wants to teach us.

Week 12 Day 2 | *Fruit of the Spirit: Joy*

Joy is often misunderstood. It seems simply like a decision one makes to be happy or to find the good in one's circumstances. Yet a quick examination of Scripture shows us something different.

Look what Nehemiah told the Israelites as they were weeping while listening to the words of the Law:

> *"Do not grieve, for the joy of the Lord is your strength."*
> —Nehemiah 8:10 (NIV)

The Jews stirred up persecution against Paul and Barnabas in Acts 13, banning them from the region. What was the response from Paul and Barnabas? Verses 51 and 52 say, "So they shook the dust off their feet as a warning to them and went to Iconium. And the disciples were filled with joy and with the Holy Spirit."

Peter writes in reference to Jesus, "Though you have not seen him, you love him; and even though you do not see him now, you believe in him and are filled with an inexpressible and glorious joy, for you are receiving the end result of your faith, the salvation of your souls" (1 Peter 1:8–9).

What do you notice about joy in these passages? Never once is it presented as a choice. In fact, never is it something we do on our own. For joy to be our strength, as mentioned in Nehemiah, it's the "joy of the Lord." In Acts, Paul and Barnabas were filled with joy in spite of being poorly treated. Similarly, in 1 Peter, joy came into the lives of the church . . . as the church believed in Christ. In other words, joy was a byproduct of something the Lord did. Joy was not something that simply came from anyone's own choosing.

Did you ever sing the song "Down In My Heart" in Sunday school, youth group, or maybe at church camp? If not, believe me, it's a classic children's Bible song. The first verse goes:

> *I've got the joy, joy, joy, joy*
> *Down in my heart.*
> *Where?*

Down in my heart.
Where?
Down in my heart.
I've got the joy, joy, joy, joy
Down in my heart.
Down in my heart to stay.

Now joy is one thing to sing about, but it's quite another to live it. Perhaps your joy is buried so far down in your heart, you have a hard time digging it out. Instead, you've got the *gloom, gloom, gloom, gloom, down in your heart*. Or maybe it's *grief, grief, grief, grief,* or *fear, fear, fear, fear?* Whatever restrains your joy, it weighs heavy like an anchor rather than guiding you like the wind.

However, living a joy-filled life is incredibly powerful because your circumstances become peripheral rather than dominant. The trials in your life may not get any better. In fact, they could get worse, as they did for Paul and Barnabas. Yet your reaction to your circumstances gets better because the Holy Spirit is in control and the joy of the Lord becomes your strength. Joy can be your response regardless of what's going on in your life.

The Holy Spirit can bear the fruit of joy in your life, including your fitness journey. The scale may not change. You may not get faster. You may not get as strong as you were hoping. Your clothes may not fit the way you'd like. Nevertheless you can still have joy.

It's not the results of your fitness that brings God glory. It's the process of depending on the Holy Spirit that brings God glory. That same process, consequently, results in experiencing more joy.

You must rely on who the Holy Spirit is and what He can do, rather than who you are and what you can't. When you rely on the Holy Spirit, you are relying on His strength. When you rely on His strength, you will find you not only enjoy life more, but you enjoy God more. Enjoying God naturally culminates in experiencing more joy.

Prayer

Father, thank You for the incredible gift of joy. Will You forgive me when I try to manufacture it myself? Please help me to rely solely on Your perfect Holy Spirit to bear much fruit in every area of my life. Amen.

Meditation

I can be joyful because of your joy in me.

Daily Spiritual Exercise

Today you will focus on the fruit of joy. Remember, these are not "fruits of ourselves." These are the outcomes of the Holy Spirit working in and through our lives.

As you are focusing on the fruit of joy, pray for wisdom. You may need help in discerning whether you're working out of your efforts or allowing the Holy Spirit to work.

Also, be sure to be teachable. Sometimes we are being taught a lesson we don't want to learn. If we are truly open to the Lord working in our lives, however, we need to humbly receive all He wants to teach us.

Week 12 Day 3 | *Fruit of the Spirit: Faithfulness*

Noticed how the farther you get from the pain of a moment, the more likely you are to repeat whatever caused it? Ever been sitting in a dentist chair getting a needle shoved in your gums so that a cavity can be fixed? You probably think to yourself, "I'm going to brush, floss, and mouthwash daily for the rest of my life!" Later that night, sure enough, you do all three. You even do it the next night, and maybe the night after. However, later that week or the next, things shift a little. It's late one night. You're tired and you've done pretty well up until now. Surely missing one night of flossing won't hurt you, so you just gargle and brush. Then, you skip the floss and the gargle the next night. Settling for a quick brush, you say you'll start fresh on Monday. Before you know it, flossing and gargling are once again the exception, not the rule—at least until your next cavity.

Pain can be a good teacher, but it can also have a short memory. This is especially true with fitness. You can work your tail off getting in shape for the summer. You suffer through one pitiful workout after another, braving a thousand salads and drinking more water than you thought possible. The process can be miserable and you swear to yourself you'll never let yourself get out of shape again. It's just too hard getting back to where you once were or where you want to be.

You stick with it, though, and what do you know? June comes around and you've gotten some results—great results, in fact. You feel fantastic, perhaps even celebratory. Maybe you deserve a week off from working out, a few nights out to enjoy some treat meals, or both! One week turns into a week and a half. A one-time celebration becomes a weekly event. You may not totally fall off the wagon, but you're not exactly riding shotgun all the time either. By the time autumn rolls around, your previous fitness high is on a downward trend. Come winter, you're back to where you were.

The good news is that your life doesn't have to be characterized in this way. I'm not talking about only using the self-discipline the Holy Spirit works in us. We already talked about that. I'm talking about loyalty. I'm talking about consistency. I'm talking about faithfulness. Mind you, we aren't relying on our faithfulness. It's not up to us to merely gut it out.

That's why it's called a fruit "of the Spirit." It's the Holy Spirit who will be faithful for us, to us, in us, and through us.

Ultimately, honoring God with our bodies is not only about avoiding pain. It's also about embracing power. God sent His Holy Spirit to work in your life. The Lord wants to draw you close to Him. To get you more reliant on Him. To make you more like Him.

Why is it important to be like Him? Because He is faithful!

> *"For the word of the Lord is right and true; he is faithful in all he does."—Psalm 33:4 (NIV)*

The more we are like the Lord by obeying the Holy Spirit working in our lives, the more faithful we become.

Fortunately for us, God's faithfulness does not depend on us:

> *"If we are faithless, he remains faithful, for he cannot disown himself."—2 Timothy 2:13 (NIV)*

He remains faithful even when we do not. This is not a license to botch it on purpose, but rather a testament to His character . . . the same character the Holy Spirit is shaping in you.

You are a little more than a week away from being finished with this 13-week journey. In order to keep your fitness going, you'll want to hold fast to the fruit of faithfulness of the Holy Spirit by following Him in simple obedience. Submit daily to His leading and He will grow the fruit of faithfulness in your life.

Make no mistake; you can be faithful in this because He is faithful in you. He is faithful not so you can show off in a bathing suit. He is faithful in you so that you might shine a light on His name, that He would be glorified:

> *"Not to us, Lord, not to us but to your name be the glory, because of your love and faithfulness."—Psalm 115:1 (NIV)*

The Holy Spirit's faithfulness does not ebb and flow. If your ability to remain faithful starts slipping, then it's likely you are working out of your own strength. You can be consistent in your fitness by relying on the faithful prompting He provides and following in obedience.

Faithfulness brings better fitness results and more importantly, more glory to the Father.

Prayer

Father, thank You for promising to be faithful to us and in us by the working of the Holy Spirit. Will You forgive me when I rely on my own strength? Please help me be more reliant on Your power in me to stay the course every day. Amen.

Meditation

I can be faithful by relying on Your faithfulness in me.

Daily Spiritual Exercise

Today you will focus on the fruit of faithfulness. Remember, these are not "fruits of ourselves." These are the outcomes of the Holy Spirit working in and through our lives.

As you are focusing on the fruit of faithfulness, pray for wisdom. You may need help in discerning whether you're working out of your efforts or allowing the Holy Spirit to work.

Also, be sure to be teachable. Sometimes we are being taught a lesson we don't want to learn. If we are truly open to the Lord working in our lives however, we need to humbly receive all that He wants to teach us.

Week 12 Day 4 | *Fruit of the Spirit: Patience*

When we talk about patience, we typically categorize it in one of three ways. Most commonly, we think of patience in terms of *how we wait for something to happen*. When we are excited about a trip, we have a hard time being patient for it to begin. When children want something, they can be impatient as they wait. We are eager for fitness results and have a hard time when they don't come as quickly as we want. Most often, dealing with patience is merely *waiting on the future*.

We also think of patience in terms of *dealing with the behavior of other people*: "They really tried my patience!" We complain to our spouse or friends after a hard day. Our children's or a roommate's actions can be taxing on our ability to deal with them in a calm, productive manner. Even the performance of our favorite sports teams can cause undue anxiety, as we root for their success. Enduring these kinds of situations can often be harder than waiting on the future.

Waiting is linear, actually requiring very little from us. Behavioral patience, on the other hand, requires an internal response (something we can control) to an external action from someone else (something we can't control).

Another way to think of patience is in terms of God's timing. This is really a combination of the first two forms of patience. It requires *waiting on a future event in which we've specifically asked for God's involvement*—His "behavior," if you will. Take, for instance, when I was single. Waiting for God to bring Kim into my life took spiritual and emotional maturing in my life.

There are many examples of waiting for God. When we pray for the salvation of family or a friend, we have to experience a different kind of patience. When we ask God for direction with a ministry opportunity, or seeking wisdom for a business venture, or praying for the return of Jesus Christ—all these require this third kind of patience: waiting on the Lord.

Yet there's a type of patience that usually goes unexamined: *patience with ourselves*. We know we need to have more patience waiting, with the behavior of others or with God's timing. That's not the same as having patience with ourselves.

Having patience with yourself is a key factor in your ability to grow spiritually and emotionally. It certainly helps with your fitness. Too often, however, we will extend patience to everyone except to ourselves. For example, was there ever a school subject that had certain aspects you struggled with grasping? Perhaps math wasn't your strong suit. The fundamentals made sense. Then, the teacher started including letters in the problems instead of just numbers . . . and your brain exploded. You didn't understand it the first, second, or tenth time. Quickly, you deemed yourself dumb.

Maybe you're trying a new discipline and it's just not sinking in. My wife is gifted at many things; however, cooking is not one of them. (She has given me permission to say this, by the way). She's made great strides. Even still, sometimes ingredients accidentally get left out of the recipe and she feels like a failure. Or, maybe she's followed the recipe perfectly but it's just not a family favorite. Rather than blaming the recipe, she blames herself . . . giving herself no grace and offering herself no patience. It makes me sad when I see her beat herself up over it. In fact, whenever we fail to be patient with ourselves, it affects those around us on some level. We don't like seeing people hurting, perhaps especially when their pain originates from messages they're telling themselves.

An amazing benefit of improved fitness is that it helps you improve emotionally as much as it does physically. As you get stronger or faster or lighter or whatever, you grow emboldened, empowered, and confident. You get emotionally stronger. The path to that kind of growth, however, requires patience with yourself. When you can barely do five pushups, what internal message will you tell yourself? When you cave on your nutrition, what voice will you hear? Or when you start an exercise program or eating regimen over and over for the umpteenth time? Will you approach it from a place of doubt or will you give yourself room to grow from your previous defeats? Your ability to be patient with yourself will help determine the outcome.

What's interesting about patience is the degree of helplessness we feel when we're trying to exercise it. We can't speed up time. We can't control other people's behavior. We can't mess with God's calendar. Our knee-jerk reaction to our own personal failures is part of living in a fallen world.

However, God wants us to recognize our helplessness when it comes to being patient! Our failure moves us away from relying on ourselves and moves us toward relying on Him.

The more we rely on Him, the more fruit we bear. That fruit is powerful, able to develop patience, including patience with ourselves:

> *"May you be strengthened with all power, according to his glorious might, for all endurance and patience with joy . . ."*
> *—Colossians 1:11 (ESV)*

We aren't supposed to rely on ourselves, because apart from Him we can do no good thing. So, accepting our helplessness is healthy! It presents us with a great opportunity to be humbly obedient. We can rely on the Holy Spirit to empower our lives, trusting God to take care of the results.

Furthermore, as you depend on the Holy Spirit to bear fruit, remember that the Lord has been patient with you. Who, then, are you not to be patient with yourself?

The Holy Spirit is more than able to bear the fruit of patience in your life: patience with the future, patience with others, patience with God, and patience with yourself. Just remember, God's timetable is not our timetable. Allow Him to slow you down so that you can recognize His providence. When you do, He will strengthen you to endure in your fitness and your faith.

Prayer

Father, thank You for the incredible amount of patience You have shown me throughout my life. Will You forgive me when I am impatient with others, with myself, and worst of all, with You? Please help me always rely on Your Holy Spirit within me to work Your will for my life. Amen.

Meditation

I will trust that the Holy Spirit will produce patience in me.

Daily Spiritual Exercise

Today you will focus on the fruit of patience. Remember, these are not "fruits of ourselves." These are the outcomes of the Holy Spirit working in and through our lives.

As you are focusing on the fruit of patience, pray for wisdom. You may need help in discerning whether you're working out of your efforts or allowing the Holy Spirit to work.

Also, be sure to be teachable. Sometimes we are being taught a lesson we don't want to learn. If we are truly open to the Lord working in our lives, however, we need to humbly receive all He wants to teach us.

Week 12 Day 5 | *Fruit of the Spirit: Peace*

When have you felt the most at peace? If you're like a lot of people, peace ebbs and flows according to what's going on in your life.

Maybe you noticed you had the most peace after completing a major project at work. Perhaps you had a huge sense of calm after paying off your student loans. Peace might have come when you had your first baby or when you held your grandchild after your daughter's difficult delivery. It could be a little daily dose of tranquility, but only after surviving a workout you didn't want to do. Fighting through the temptation of junk food cravings can bring peace too.

There are a few problems with this kind of peace. First of all, it's more akin to relief than true peace. You're experiencing a reprieve from a heavy workload, stressful situation, financial pressure, or temptation. The heaviness of the burden has been lifted. You feel you can now breathe, but it correlates to the lack of trouble you're facing.

Since it's related to a specific issue, that emotion is circumstantial. When things are going well, you feel "peace." However, when things are hard, frustrating, and fear-filled, there is no harmony. The events in your life dictate when you experience peace.

Of course, if the peace you know is circumstantial, then it's temporary. It's only around for as long as the pressures are absent. When one trial is resolved, the inner stillness returns. Then a new trouble arises and the peace is gone once again. Temporary peace is really no kind of peace at all. Even when things seem at ease, in the back of your mind you know it won't last. That causes a spirit of unrest. Peace and unrest cannot coexist.

The Holy Spirit bears the fruit of peace, unlike the conditional, fleeting kind we have come to know. His peace is rooted in a permanent, saving relationship with Jesus Christ. That transcends any kind of earthly peace we might claim.

Unlike relief, true peace will allow you to breathe all the time. Rather than an absence of heaviness, there's freedom even amid heaviness.

That's because it's not coming from the removal of something hard.

Peace, the fruit of the Holy Spirit, is unlike earthly peace. It is unrelated to what's going on in our lives. It doesn't depend on us to perform, produce, achieve, or avoid. It's unrelated to anything we do because it's Christ working through us. His peace has the power not only to withstand the hard times, but to triumph in them.

Also, the Holy Spirit's peace is permanent. True peace is built upon a relationship with Jesus Christ; therefore, it's steadfast and dependable. It doesn't ebb and flow. It's trustworthy and faithful and can characterize our lives not just at certain times, but *at all times.*

Towards the end of a fitness journey such as ours, people are usually feeling one of the following emotions: 1) This has been awful. I haven't gotten near the results I had hoped. I'll never get there. 2) I saw some results in the beginning, but then I slacked off. Now I'm back to where I was. What should I try next? 3) This has been good, but I just don't think I can keep it up. 4) This has been awesome. I sure hope I don't lose my mojo.

All of these outcomes incorporate the man-made, performance-based kind of peace, but it doesn't have to be that way. No matter what kind of physical results you've seen, the Holy Spirit can produce His perfect peace in your life.

Here's the blueprint:

> *"Don't worry about anything; instead, pray about everything. Tell God what you need, and thank him for all he has done. Then you will experience God's peace, which exceeds anything we can understand. His peace will guard your hearts and minds as you live in Christ Jesus."—Philippians 4:6–7 (NLT)*

First thing, don't worry. Don't be anxious. That's not the same as saying, "Do nothing about it." Rather, while you're working on your fitness, don't get caught up in the emotional highs and lows of your progress. Don't give your fitness that kind of power.

Then, you pray about it. You can pray about everything. Last time I checked, fitness is part of "everything." While you are praying, you can tell God what you need. At the top of the list of what you need should be a clean heart and pure motives, that you might bring Him glory.

Lastly, you should be dependent on Him for all things. As such, you should always make known your appreciation for what He's done, for the answers He has given you. You want to show God gratitude in all situations, regardless of the outcome.

Look at what happens! You can and will experience "God's peace," which far exceeds the earthly peace you might try to manufacture. It will keep you safe as it guards you. *The Living Bible* translates it as, "His peace will keep your thoughts and your hearts quiet and at rest . . ."

Quiet thoughts and a heart at rest—this is true peace. The kind that can be experienced no matter how difficult or disappointing the situation. The kind of peace that surpasses understanding. The kind given by our Everlasting Father . . . the Prince of Peace.

If you keep the Father at the center of your fitness, you can be at peace regardless of the results. That's because God's peace is always available to His children as a fruit of the Holy Spirit. His peace will produce contentment without producing complacency, a perfect balance able to sustain you in your fitness pursuits.

Prayer
Father, thank You for the Holy Spirit and the peace He can produce. Will You forgive me when I worry or am thankless or fail to pray? Please help me to rest always in the gift of the cross. Amen.

Meditation
The peace produced by the Holy Spirit can characterize my life.

Daily Spiritual Exercise
Today you will focus on the fruit of peace. Remember, these are not "fruits of ourselves." These are the outcomes of the Holy Spirit working in and through our lives.

As you are focusing on the fruit of peace, pray for wisdom. You may need help in discerning whether you're working out of your efforts or allowing the Holy Spirit to work.

Also, be sure to be teachable. Sometimes we are being taught a lesson we don't want to learn. If we are truly open to the Lord working in our lives, however, we need to humbly receive all He wants to teach us.

Week 12 Day 6 | *Fruit of the Spirit: Gentleness*

Gentleness is a misunderstood quality. We tend to think of someone who is gentle as merely being "kind" and "sweet." Certainly, gentleness requires a sense of kindness, but kindness and sweetness do not necessarily conclude in gentleness. In fact, gentleness as a fruit of the Spirit isn't even likely what you think.

A better translation for gentleness in this context would probably be "meekness." So, from now on, when you think about the fruit of gentleness, think of meekness.

To make matters even more confusing, meekness isn't likely what you think, either. If we are to truly understand the fruit of gentleness, we must also understand meekness.

Meekness gets a bad rap. If I said someone was meek, you would probably think they were "timid" or "weak," or both. With that understanding, we misinterpret the beatitude, "Blessed are the meek, for they shall inherit the earth" (Matthew 5:5). Admit it: reading that beatitude makes you think that a strong, assertive person will not inherit the earth. The reward is reserved for the opposite type of personality, the timid or weak.

The Greeks, however, defined meekness as "strength or power under control." Sound like anyone you know? Jesus, maybe? He had legions of angels at His disposal (Matthew 26:53). He could turn water into wine (John 2:7–9) or walk on water (Matthew 14:25) at will. He had the ability to heal the sick, fix the broken, and conquer death (Matthew 11:5). Jesus was the epitome of power under control. There was nothing feeble about Jesus. He was meek.

So, what other attributes comprise meekness? Certainly, humility is one. Romans 12:3 tells us not to think too highly of ourselves. When we do, we are unteachable. The unteachable are the unreachable. A humble heart, however, can be molded and used for His glory.

Meekness also requires submissiveness. We're to remain open to the Lord's leading in our lives and the imparting of His Word into our hearts. Then, we can live in the transformative power of Christ working through us.

Graciousness is an underlying characteristic of meekness. Look at how Philippians 4:5 uses the word "let" rather than "make" when talking about the cousin of meekness, gentleness:

> *"Let your gentleness be evident to all. The Lord is near."*
> *—Philippians 4:5 (NIV)*

If I were to say kindly, "Will you let the dog out, please," there's a sense of natural cordiality in the process. Now if I said, "Make the dog go out," that graciousness is gone. In the same way, we don't "make" our gentleness known. We "let" it be known. That requires a graciousness that arises out of the Holy Spirit in us.

Okay, so meekness is a combined result of the Spirit exhibiting power, humility, submissiveness, and graciousness in our lives. That's great, but what's that have to do with fitness?

Nearly 12 weeks of this fitness journey are completed. If you've been diligent, you've likely experienced one or both of the following situations.

The first situation we talked about briefly when we covered Job and his unsupportive friend base. There's a chance that your efforts to be healthier have unintentionally convicted some people around you about their own health. However, rather than talking to you about it in a productive manner, something else happens. Out of their insecurities or lack of understanding, they have discouraged, doubted, teased, or tempted you with their careless remarks. During times like these, you'll quickly learn whether the fruit of gentleness is evident in your life. Responding in kind or wilting under their words displays a lack of controlled strength.

We have Paul and Timothy to encourage us:

> *"Bear with each other and forgive one another if any of you has a grievance against someone. Forgive as the Lord forgave you."*
> *—Colossians 3:13 (NIV)*

This is a whole lot easier if we first clothe ourselves in gentleness, as we're instructed in verse 12.

The other situation you may find yourself in is wanting to "help" others with all your newfound knowledge and expertise. You've been so successful, you now have the urge to generously share your discoveries with the world, letting everyone bask in and learn from the greatness of your achievement. Now, wanting to help others with their fitness can come from an authentic and loving place in your heart. It can also come from the desire for attention, accolades, and feedback. Are we "letting" our gentleness be known? Or, with a lack of humility that we might not see, are we "making" our abilities known, as we attempt to impress others?

Paul is there for us again, and again, with the same remedy:

> *"Be completely humble and gentle; be patient, bearing with one another in love."—Ephesians 4:2 (NIV)*

Whether it is insensitivities to your fitness ambitions or a friend's lack of fitness ambitions, gentleness and meekness are required. As my parents are fond of saying, "Whatever God requires, He provides." In this case, like so many others, He provided the Holy Spirit, and the Holy Spirit can produce gentleness and meekness in you.

Remember, gentleness and meekness are produced out of strength. That strength needs to come from the Holy Spirit or it won't be sustainable. Be strong in the Lord by recognizing that your reliance on Him is no weakness at all.

Prayer
Father, thank You for giving us Jesus as the ultimate example of power, humility, submissiveness, and graciousness. Will You forgive me when I let my arrogance or defensiveness win out? Please help me live a life characterized by gentleness and meekness. Amen.

Meditation
Let Your gentleness with me manifest in gentleness through me.

Daily Spiritual Exercise

Today you will focus on the fruit of gentleness. Remember, these are not "fruits of ourselves." These are the outcomes of the Holy Spirit working in and through our lives.

As you are focusing on the fruit of gentleness, pray for wisdom. You may need help in discerning whether you're working out of your efforts or allowing the Holy Spirit to work.

Also, be sure to be teachable. Sometimes we are being taught a lesson we don't want to learn. If we are truly open to the Lord working in our lives, however, we need to humbly receive all He wants to teach us.

Week 12 Day 7 | *Fruit of the Spirit: Goodness*

To understand how "goodness" can help us with our fitness, we first need to better understand what it is exactly. Coming from the Greek word *agathos*, goodness is moral and spiritual excellence. Now, that sounds a little boring until we take a look at the goodness of God's nature. There we'll quickly get excited at the prospect of the Spirit bearing this same fruit in our lives.

God's goodness **protects** (Psalm 34:7; Psalm 86:17; Psalm 109:21) and His goodness **provides** (Psalm 34:9–10).

His goodness **renews** us (Psalm 119:40) and it **rescues** us (Psalm 116:12; Psalm 142:7).

His goodness **saves** (Psalm 96:2) and it **liberates** (Psalm 129:4).

His goodness is **mercy** (Psalm 116:5), a mercy so good that it **forgives** (Psalm 86:5), **forgets** (Micah 7:19), and **instructs** (Psalm 25:7–9)

His news is good (Matthew 9:35; Mark 1:15) and **His name** is good (Psalm 54:6).

His word is good (Hebrews 6:4–6) and **His will** is good (Romans 12:2).

His judgment, (Psalm 119:66), **His laws** (Psalm 119:39), and even **His disciplines** (Psalm 119:67–71; Isaiah 38:16; Hebrews 12:10) are all good.

His gifts are good (James 1:17; Matthew 7:11) and those good gifts are **abundant** (Psalm 31:19) because **His goodness is abundant** (Psalm 145:7). And of course, **His love** is good (Psalm 69:16).

So together, His love and His goodness are available to us. Not only that, but they are pursuing us all the time, for all of our life:

> *"Surely your goodness and love will follow me all the days of my life, and I will dwell in the house of the Lord forever."—Psalm 23:6 (NIV)*

Excited yet?

It's out of His goodness that He gave us bodies that move, eat, and sleep. Yet the temptation is to look at exercise, eating healthy, and getting sufficient sleep as sacrifices, not privileges. Far too often, we dread working out rather than being grateful for able bodies equipped to do amazing things. These amazing things benefit us, by the way.

Out of the goodness of His plan for our bodies, when we exercise, we release "feel good" hormones called endorphins. Out of that same goodness, when we exercise, our bodies get healthier, which makes life easier. Out of His goodness, healthier bodies help us feel better, have more confidence, do more, and enjoy more.

Yet, we tend to dread exercise, a good gift that keeps on giving. The same can be said of eating healthy and getting adequate rest. We prioritize other things at the expense of enjoying the blessings He's orchestrated out of the goodness of His nature. It's not that we want too much; it's that we're settling for too little.

It doesn't have to be this way. We can enjoy our fitness. We can look forward to a workout. We can enjoy healthy food and have bodies nourished by solid sleep. This is good news if you're still struggling with enjoying any or all parts of honoring God with your body. Start praying that out of the goodness of His character, He will change you—that He would renew your outlook, that you could rely on the fruit of His goodness working out of you to provide that change.

The Holy Spirit wants you to rely on Him for all things. For your fitness. For your comfort. For your heart, mind, attitude, and of course, for your goodness. The only way goodness is manifested in your life is when it originates from and is empowered by the Holy Spirit as He leads and guides. So, if you are ever going to add goodness to your faithfulness (2 Peter 1:5), it must come as a fruit of the Holy Spirit.

Yet once again, in His perfect goodness, God's plan comes full circle. The Spirit we need is the Spirit He provides, and that Spirit is good too:

"Teach me to do your will, for you are my God; may your good
Spirit lead me on level ground."—Psalm 143:10 (NIV)

Living a Holy Spirit–powered life requires us to recognize God's pure, perfect goodness. Out of that goodness, He can enable us to enjoy our fitness by first enjoying Him.

If you're struggling with your fitness, focus first on enjoying God's goodness demonstrated throughout your life. My guess is that you'll soon realize that the Holy Spirit's fruit of goodness isn't just good; it's great (Psalm 31:19).

Prayer
Father, thank You for your immeasurable goodness. Will You please forgive me when I rely on myself to produce the change I need? Please help me to always focus on the fruit of Your goodness toward me and working in me. Amen.

Meditation
The fruit of your goodness can change me.

Daily Spiritual Exercise
Today you will focus on the fruit of goodness. Remember, these are not "fruits of ourselves." These are the outcomes of the Holy Spirit working in and through our lives.

As you are focusing on the fruit of goodness, pray for wisdom. You may need help in discerning whether you're working out of your efforts or allowing the Holy Spirit to work.

Also, be sure to be teachable. Sometimes we are being taught a lesson we don't want to learn. If we are truly open to the Lord working in our lives, however, we need to humbly receive all He wants to teach us.

WEEK 13 PREVIEW

Names for You

Here we are . . . the final week of our 13-week fitness journey. Day 85, to be exact. You've likely learned a lot about yourself over the course of these weeks.

You've learned what kind of exercises you like, what kind you don't, those you're good at, and those you aren't.

You've probably tried some new foods, implemented new nutritional goals, increased your water intake, or decreased your junk food intake. If so, you've seen what a profound effect nutrition can have on your fitness level.

I also hope you've discovered the valuable role sleep plays in your overall fitness. Not only does sleep help your body repair and prepare physiologically, you'll be better equipped psychologically for your day. You'll be better able to make the right decisions concerning your exercise and nutrition.

Aside from the physical lessons you've learned, my prayer is that you've discovered even more about yourself spiritually. I hope you've developed a great appreciation for what our God has done for us. Then, out of that gratitude, you feel compelled to bring Him glory and honor . . . mind, body, and spirit.

We've looked at Old and New Testament heroes who've modeled extraordinary faith and who saw victory in the face of defeat. We've seen how to be equipped with the full armor of God, which gives us great freedom to run a race that He's already won.

We focused on the unbreakable promises God has for us throughout Scripture. If we cling to and rely on God and His promises, He will produce life-changing fruit in our lives. We've examined the persons of Jesus, God the Father, and the Holy Spirit.

The God of all creation has sent his King Son to save us. The Lord then imparted the perfect Holy Spirit to work in our lives as we live by His strength. We should be encouraged!

Unfortunately, we don't always live a Spirit-filled, Spirit-focused life. Oftentimes, the temptation is to look at Scripture through a lens of generality rather than specificity. It's kind of like knowing you play for the best sports team in the country. Your team is rich in history and success. Your coach has all the credentials and has proven himself trustworthy time and time again. You're surrounded by teammates with astounding skills and a proven track record. You know the plays by heart and watched film on the opposing team, and your team has a winning record. No other team comes close. So you know that ultimately, you can't lose.

Yet, in spite of all these things, you still feel like an outsider. You still feel like all these advantages apply to everyone on the team—and maybe on our fitness journey—*except* you. In your mind, it seems these things are *generally* right . . . for everyone else. Somehow, though, they don't or can't *specifically* apply to you. After all, you know yourself pretty well and you just don't see yourself that way . . . as victorious.

Does this sound like you, even after 12 weeks of examining the kind of encouragement and assurances we've been given? If so, this week should help. This week we're going to look at what the God of the Bible has to say specifically about you—at who you are because of Him. At what you are because of Him. At what you can do because of Him.

Life changes when we see ourselves the way our loving Father sees us. Then we can better align our minds with His mind. Then we can better align our spirit with His Spirit. Then we can experience true triumph. When our minds and spirits are experiencing victory, it makes it far easier for our bodies to follow suit.

It's a lot easier to see how magnificent our God is than it is seeing any good in us. That is, until we start looking at ourselves through His eyes. When we see us the way He sees us, when we start listening to what He says about us, we start feeling empowered to live the magnificent life He created us to live.

Daily Spiritual Exercise: Because of Christ, I am _____.

For each of the next six days, we'll look at a name or description that God has given you. Write it down. Next to it, write down the implications it will have in your life—what it will enable you to accomplish, how it affects your struggles, and/or how it equips you for victory. Post it somewhere you can see it regularly. Every time you do, ask the Lord to help you believe it. Pray that He will help you to see yourself the way He does.

Week 13 Day 1 | *Names for You: Conqueror*

Is your memory good enough to remember the test-taking days when you were in school? Depending on how well you prepared, you had one of three perceptions of your performance.

If you barely studied or had a hard time with the material? You'd turn in the test with a sinking feeling, knowing it would not go well for you. You bombed it.

If you spent a good amount of time reviewing your notes and had a decent grasp on most of it? You might turn in the test thinking, "Not awful, but I'm glad it's over." You survived it.

Or maybe you took great notes, understood the material frontwards and backwards, and had little trouble on test day? What a great feeling . . . you aced it!

The feeling of acing tests was infinitely better than bombing them. Doing well was also more empowering than merely surviving the test. You felt strengthened and liberated because you had mastered the test topic and it held no power over you. Because of your diligence and hard work, you conquered that test!

As we near the end of our 90-day fitness journey, you're likely feeling one of those same three ways: you bombed it, survived it, or aced it.

Romans 8 is an amazing chapter filled with encouragement, hope, and power that can speak truth into our lives regardless of how the fitness journey is going.

We are encouraged by verses 1–17 as they remind us of the freedom we have living through the Spirit. How encouraging that we're not slaves to sin. We belong to Christ. By His Spirit working in us, we are free to live lives that glorify Him. We have victory!

As verses 18–30 tells us, we also have hope. Whatever pain and suffering we are going through now (including the suffering, frustration, and disappointment if we "bombed" another attempt to get fit), all of it will pale in comparison to the glory that awaits us. There's also hope in the meantime because the Spirit is here to help us amid our weakness. We have hope for our lives, both now and for the day when God's glory is fully revealed. That hope leaves us victorious again.

Verses 31–39 encourage us about God's great power and what Jesus did for us on the cross. Through Him, we can have a relationship with God that is insurmountable, unbeatable, and inseparable. That's powerful and it's another victory!

When we partake in victory after victory after victory, we are, by definition, conquerors. No matter how you think your fitness journey is going, you are a conqueror. Whether you're getting faster, stronger, lighter, heavier, healthier, fitter, or not, you are a conqueror.

Actually, we aren't mere conquerors . . . we are *more* than that:

> "No, in all these things we are more than conquerors through him who loved us."—Romans 8:37

More than conquerors—that's how God sees us. That's what we are.

There's even more good news! Unlike taking a test where it all depends on your efforts, being more than a conqueror is independent of you! It's all "through him who loved us." God loves us with a love that "neither death nor life, neither angels nor demons, neither the present nor the future, nor any powers, neither height nor depth, nor anything else in all creation, will be able to separate us from."

Through our relationship with Christ, there is no obstacle or trial or situation that He cannot triumph over. The resulting victories are for our good and His glory.

If we can't be separated from a love that can't be overcome, victory is not only possible; it's assured. Assured victories are the hallmark of those who are more than a conqueror.

That someone is you.

Prayer

Father, thank You for the encouragement, hope, and power we find in Romans 8. Will You forgive me when I'm looking inward and focused on my own efforts? Please help me to see myself as more than a conqueror through Your eyes, not because of anything I've done, but only from the victory we have in Your Son. Amen.

Meditation

Because of You, I am more than a conqueror.

Daily Spiritual Exercise

Romans 8:37 calls you "more than a conqueror." Get out a sheet of paper and write down, "Because of Christ, I am more than a conqueror." Next to it, write down the implications this has in your life—what it will enable you to accomplish, how it affects your struggles, how it equips you for victory.

Post it someplace where you can see it regularly. Every time you do, ask the Lord to help you believe it. Pray that He will help you to see yourself the way He does. Give Him praise when He does.

Week 13 Day 2 | *Names for You: Citizen*

For our honeymoon, my wife and I were blessed to go to Aruba. If you are unfamiliar, it's a very small island in the Caribbean Sea, just north of Venezuela.

This was my first trip out of the country and I wasn't exactly sure what to expect. Of course, the brochures made it look amazing and the reviews sounded wonderful. Still, it was far from home and from anything familiar. To get there, we needed plane tickets, reservations, proof of identification, and a passport. In order to get the passport, I needed my birth certificate. I also needed my driver's license, which originally required my Social Security card. Those credentials not only proved that I was who I said I was, they guaranteed various rights and privileges I had as an American.

Well, Aruba was fantastic. The water was crystal clear. The trade winds provided a welcome relief from the hot sun. The people were warm and accommodating . . . true to the claim of being "One Happy Island." We had a great time and didn't want it to end.

The strange thing is that it was hard to feel like we belonged there. I'm not sure if it was because it didn't seem real . . . or whether it was too good to be true. It didn't seem we really had the right to be there in the first place. Aruba certainly wasn't our island. We could claim none of the rights and privileges afforded to the natives. Yes, we were taken care of, but we were taken care of as guests. That's just a nicer way for the resort to describe an outsider. The inherent sense of home, familiarity, and nationality would not be restored until we stepped foot back on American soil.

For Christians, the Bible paints a very different picture of heaven than how I felt in Aruba:

> *"Now you are no longer strangers to God and foreigners to heaven, but you are members of God's very own family, citizens of God's country, and you belong in God's household with every other Christian."–Ephesians 2:19 (TLB)*

Wow! Don't gloss over the power and comfort Paul is giving us here.

The Bible says we are no longer strangers to God, or as The Message puts it, "wandering exiles." We once were alienated because of our sin, but no more. Instead of being strangers to God, as we were in the past, we have a relationship with God now, one that will make us residents of heaven in the future.

We have a new citizenship, a citizenship in God's country. The Message says it like this: "This kingdom of faith is now your home country." In a sense, we have been given a new nationality based on faith and our eternal identification with Christ. No Social Security card, birth certificate, passport, or driver's license required.

What does this mean for our fitness? We have the *right* to come to God with our struggles and lay them before Him. We have the *honor* of approaching our fitness as another means to bring our King glory. We have the *freedom* to enjoy using our earthly bodies and the *privilege* of getting new, perfect bodies in heaven.

You're a citizen with all the rights, honors, freedoms, and privileges that come with belonging in God's household.

We were not made for this world. Our heavenly citizenship gives us hope for our future, while empowering us to live a victorious life on earth.

The perfect citizenship in a perfect Heaven with a perfect God for a perfect eternity—what could be better?

Prayer
Father, thank You for making me a citizen. Forgive me when I set my mind on an earthly citizenship rather than one with You. Please help me to always remember that my home is in Heaven. Because of that, I have the freedom to approach You with anything while here on earth. Amen.

Meditation
My citizenship is in heaven.

Daily Spiritual Exercise

Ephesians 2:19 reminds us of our heavenly heritage. Get out a sheet of paper and write down, "Because of Christ, I am a citizen of heaven." Next to it, write down the implications this has in your life —what it will enable you to accomplish, how it affects your struggles, how it equips you for victory.

Then, post it somewhere you can see it regularly. Every time you do, ask the Lord to help you believe it. Pray that He will help you to see yourself the way He does. Give Him praise when He does.

Week 13 Day 3 | *Names for You: Child*

My son Silas is three years old and he's a pure delight. He's a well-mannered, smiley little fellow who talks well and is generally very chipper. He's also at that age where he's really into me. I have to say, I love it. Where I go, he goes. If I'm working, he wants to work. If I have to run an errand, he wants to go. If I'm reading a devotional, he'll "read" his. He talks to me in the shower, wakes me up in the morning, and interrupts my trips to the potty. He even likes to exercise when I exercise. One morning, literally the first thing he said to me was, "Daddy, time to beast up?" He's my shadow. He adores me and I adore him.

Something else I love about Silas is that he comes to me when he needs help. Now, not everything is truly a "need." Sometimes he already knows what to do and how to do it.

"Daddy! Need help with high chair." "No, Silas, you can do it. Just keep pushing." "I can't open door, Daddy." "Yeah, you can, Silas. I've shown you what to do. Just pull down on the handle. You got it."

Other times, though, the need is real: he needs genuine help, or he's hurt, or he's scared. As his father, it's my joy and privilege to be there for him. I want him to come to me. Can't get your shoes fastened? Come to me . . . I'll help you. Fall down and bump your knee? Come to me . . . I'll kiss it. Scared of the Chick-fil-A cow? Come to me . . . I'll hold you.

This is the same relationship you are blessed to have with God because He is your heavenly Father. You are his precious child.

> *"See how very much our Father loves us, for he calls us his children, and that is what we are!"—1 John 3:1 (NLT)*

Just think about that for a moment. The God of all creation is your Father. That means you are a member of His family and belong in His household. You'll participate in the glory of His heavenly kingdom someday. Yet, you have all the benefits and advantages of being a member of His family while here on earth, now. So, you can approach Him anytime, anywhere, with anything. You can follow Him day and night.

You can be His shadow.

He wants you to come to Him, not just day or night, but day *and* night. He wants you to seek Him first, with all things and in all things. In so doing, His perfect love can spread over you like the shadow of His perfect wings:

> *"How precious is your unfailing love, O God! All humanity finds shelter in the shadow of your wings."*—Psalm 36:7 (NLT)

As His children, our Father wants us to come to Him with all things. Shouldn't that include our fitness? We can approach Him in our weakness and ask Him to make us strong: "Father, I hate exercising. I know I need to do it, but I'm struggling and I feel stuck. Can you help?"

"Lord, I've been teased, mocked, looked down upon for my weight and it really hurts. I don't want to find my worth in the eyes of man, but I do. I need Your help."

"Father, I know I shouldn't go to food for comfort because it just makes matters worse, but it's hard. Will You help?"

"God, I'm currently doing a great job of honoring You with my body, but I'm scared it won't last. Please help me."

I mentioned that sometimes I give Silas additional support and encouragement for things I know he is capable of doing. Our Father will sometimes do the same thing with us. We know the right things to do because He's already told us and shown us.

Truth be told, we just aren't willing to do them. You see, the Father always hears His children, but He doesn't always give us the answer we want as quickly as we want. He will, however, answer in the way that will ultimately bring Him the most glory. So, be honest with Him when expressing your needs because, when the need is real, He picks us up, wipes us off, kisses our scratched knees, and loves on us.

That's the Father we have: one who holds the universe in the palm of His hand, yet is tender enough to hold us in His heart.

One who is capable of handling our every need. One who said to His son, "Go to them."

One who says to us, "Come to me."

Therefore, as His children, we should go to Him, reach for His loving arms, and never stop adoring Him.

Our Heavenly Father certainly adores us.

Prayer
Father, thank You for calling me Your child. Will You forgive me when I reach for something or someone other than You? Please help me rely on the Holy Spirit for discernment and to empower me in a way that brings You joy. Amen.

Meditation
I am my Father's child.

Daily Spiritual Exercise
1 John 3:1 says that our Father calls us His children. Get out a sheet of paper and write down, "Because of Christ, I am a child of God."

Next to it, write down the implications this has in your life—what it will enable you to accomplish, how it affects your struggles, how it equips you for victory.

Then, post it somewhere you can see it regularly. Every time you do, ask the Lord to help you believe it. Pray that He will help you see yourself the way He does. Give Him praise when He does.

Week 13 Day 4 | *Names for You: Wonderfully Made*

I was watching a program recently about the so-called "Wonders of the World." It was interesting to learn about these ancient monuments and to see why and how they were built.

For instance, a Mughal emperor built the Taj Mahal in memory of his third wife at a cost of 32 million rupees (in 1648). An ornate, architectural masterpiece of reflecting pools, towers and domes, it's 240 feet high and took 20,000 workers nearly 22 years to complete.

The program also profiled the Great Wall of China. Thought to have taken 200 years to finish, it measures up to 26 feet high and 5,500 miles long. For some context, the continental United States extends about 3,000 miles from east to west. At nearly twice the length of the U.S., the Great Wall probably feels as long as this 13-week fitness journey.

Probably the prettiest and most interesting was Machu Picchu, built around 1450 by the Incas in Peru. It rises in stair-stepped grass terraces and stone retaining walls, climbing into the clouds to nearly 8,000 feet above sea level. Machu Picchu culminates in some temples, what's thought to be a clock of sorts, and glorious vistas overlooking the Urubamba Valley.

The show also took trips to Jordan to see Petra, a city carved into the stone in the side of a mountain; Christ the Redeemer, a nearly 100-foot-tall, 30-foot-wide statue in Brazil of Jesus with His arms spread wide; Chichén Itzá, a Mayan city in Mexico recognized by its ancient temples, columns, and statues; and perhaps most famous of all, the impossibly giant Great Pyramid of Giza, in Egypt, spanning 750 feet wide and 450 feet high. All, of course, are manmade, which is remarkable given the time periods in which they were constructed. These monuments took laborers and craftsmen, architects and artists, astonishing resources, time, energy, and commitment to construct.

As impressive as these structures are, however, they're all stagnant. They don't move. They don't improve. They don't grow, change, or challenge. These so called "wonders" don't think, reason, or respond. Edifices don't evolve, emote, or engage. Yes, they're impressive. Yes, they're interesting . . . that is, unless they're compared to you. On their own, the monuments are astounding . . . but next to you, they're boring.

At any given time, your body is doing trillions and trillions of things at once. Cells are dividing and reproducing. Energy sources are being consumed and replaced. Electrical impulses are firing. Light is being deciphered. Oxygen is replenishing. Germs are being battled. Muscles are moving.

Sound waves are being interpreted. Countless reactions and responses are happening constantly.

Those are only the chemical and biological reactions. Quantifying the non-physical processes is equally staggering. Thoughts produced. Problems solved. Emotions triggered. Masterpieces conceived. Ideas generated. Dreams perceived. Behaviors learned. It's astonishing when you consider what your body is capable of doing.

These amazing intricacies of our bodies were not lost on King David:

> *"You made all the delicate, inner parts of my body and knit me together in my mother's womb. Thank you for making me so wonderfully complex! Your workmanship is marvelous—how well I know it."—Psalm 139:13–14 (NLT)*

The temptation when reading this verse is to merely acknowledge the "complexity" of our bodies. We somehow gloss over the "marvelous workmanship" part. We know that there's a lot going on, things we don't understand and things we can't see. Yes, when we stop to think about it, our bodies certainly are incredible. Yet, we don't stop to think about what is happening for our bodies to sustain life. We are too focused on what we can see in the mirror. And what we can see we don't like. So, we rush past the fact that we were created by a master craftsman. The thing is, we are works of art *just as we are*. As the NIV puts it, we are "wonderfully made."

As grand as all of creation is, the Bible says we are grander still. Our creator God created only one of us, and so each of us is priceless. We are priceless, yet His Son paid the price for us, evidence of just how wonderful we are to Him.

We are closing in on the end of our 13-week journey. If you've improved your nutrition, exercised consistently, and been diligent about your sleep, you've likely seen some changes in your body, and probably in your emotions as well. You've seen His workmanship in action. You've experienced how good living can feel when you treat your body with the respect it deserves.

The challenge is this: glorifying Him with your heart . . . regardless of the results you see when you're trying to glorify Him with your body.

If you haven't seen changes, it's not an indictment of the brilliance of His craftsmanship. You are still one of a kind. You are still the work of His hands. Christ still considers you worth dying for.

Remember this always . . . there's no Wonder of the World that's made more wonderfully than you.

Prayer
Father, thank You for the incredible bodies You've crafted for us. Will You forgive me when I'm overly focused on results at the expense of overlooking what You've created? Please help me to keep You at the center of my fitness. Amen.

Meditation
I am wonderfully made by an even more wonderful Maker.

Daily Spiritual Exercise
Psalm 139:14 says you are "fearfully and wonderfully made." Get out a sheet of paper and write down, "I am wonderfully made." Next to it, write down the implications this has in your life—what it will enable you to accomplish, how it affects your struggles, how it equips you for victory.

Then, post it somewhere you can see it regularly. Every time you do, ask the Lord to help you believe it. Pray that He will help you to see yourself the way He does. Give Him praise when He does.

Week 13 Day 5 | *Names for You: Precious*

In their toddler years, our kids always enjoyed singing songs before we put them to bed. I would hold them, their heads on my shoulder, and together we'd sing some of their favorites. Of course, "Jesus Loves the Little Children" was always in the mix:

> *Jesus loves the little children*
> *All the children of the world*
> *Red and yellow, black and white*
> *They are precious in His sight*
> *Jesus loves the little children of the world.*

With their innocence, their wide-eyed faith, and inherent trust, children certainly are precious.

Somewhere along the way, we grow out of our preciousness, it would seem. Our sinful nature takes hold. We dilute the value of people, including ourselves, by overestimating things, goals, possessions, or achievements. The more worth we put on them, the more attention we give them. If they're getting too much attention, when something goes wrong, the world stops. For instance, what happens when a car nut hears a faint, muffled thud coming from the right wheel? He races to the mechanic for an immediate, state-of-the-art diagnosis.

This can happen with our fitness too. A mild injury merits an abrupt trip to the physical therapist. A panic ensues as to whether you'll set a new personal best. You become preoccupied over lost strength, so you reach for questionable supplements. An obsession with your weight has you starving yourself, leading to the numbness of indifference and defeat.

Be on guard. Matthew 6:21 says, "Wherever your treasure is, there the desires of your heart will also be." Our hobbies, possessions, and ambitions can become a little too precious to us. We can give them too much attention, treating them like treasures, giving them heart space they don't deserve.

Have you ever stopped to consider that we ourselves occupy heart space we don't deserve: the heart of our loving Father? Psalm 139 reads like a love letter from God to us, detailing the room we occupy in the heart of our Creator.

In verses 1–6, we learn that, to Him, we are precious on the inside. He cares about our hearts, our thoughts, and our words. He knows us better than we know ourselves. He knows what we will do before we do it. So, He goes ahead of us, paving a way . . . and follows behind, protecting us . . . His hands blessing us.

Next, verses 7–12 say that what happens to us is also precious to God. No matter where we go, we can't escape His Spirit. His strength supports us. There's no darkness too dark for His light to penetrate. His presence is constantly there for us to rely on . . . His hands guiding us.

Verses 13–16 show us that both our bodies and our days are precious, from His workmanship in the womb to each minute of our lives written in the book He wrote just for us—all priceless to the Author. His hands form our bodies and record our days.

Finally in verses 17–18, some of the most humbling and shocking verses of all:

> *"How precious are your thoughts about me, O God. They cannot be numbered! I can't even count them; they outnumber the grains of sand! And when I wake up, you are still with me!"—Psalm 139:17–18 (NLT)*

In spite of who we are and how we act, God thinks good things, precious things, about us. The thoughts He has of us are like treasures to Him. Like someone passionate about His treasure. He never leaves us.

Precious thoughts like endless treasures for endless days.

God treasures us so much, in fact, that He put a permanent pause in the record of human history . . . that precious space between B.C. and A.D. He sent His perfect Son, and the "precious blood of Christ" (1 Peter 1:1) was shed on the cross for the sake of His children.

Why? That we might know the Father loves us as much as He loves His Son (John 17:23).

Since we are precious, what happens to us matters to Him, especially during the trials we face. Fitness is a legitimate trial for those who've been plagued with feelings of insecurity and unworthiness their whole lives. It is no less a trial when Satan deceives us into treating our fitness like an idol.

Our trials matter because they affect our faith, and even our faith is precious to Him:

> *"These trials will show that your faith is genuine. It is being tested as fire tests and purifies gold—though your faith is far more precious than mere gold!"—1 Peter 1:7a (NLT)*

We once again see the genius and compassion of His love. God pours into us, caring for us, nurturing us, feeding us, protecting us, and providing for us. He has a relentless desire to make our value to Him evident.

We, in turn, need to repent of any sin in our lives. We submit our will. We accept His forgiveness and we rely on His strength. This faith-filled response is worth more than gold to Him!

You see, our Father doesn't just love the little children. He loves all His children.

Too often, we are our own worst critics. As such, we beat ourselves up with self-defeating, self-effacing remarks. These remarks begin to take root in our belief system, yet they're not true in the eyes of our Maker. He sees us as precious, and we would be wise to believe that about ourselves.

So, draw near to God. Hold Him close. Rest your head on His shoulders. Listen as He sings, "You are precious in My sight."

Prayer

Father, thank You for finding anything about me precious. Will You forgive me when I place too much value on the wrong things? Please help me to always place the most value on the precious blood of Your Son Jesus, and on our relationship. Amen.

Meditation

I am precious in your sight.

Daily Spiritual Exercise

Psalm 139:17 says that God thinks precious thoughts about us. Get out a sheet of paper and write down, "I am precious in the eyes of God." Next to it, write down the implications this has in your life —what it will enable you to accomplish, how it affects your struggles, how it equips you for victory.

Then, post it somewhere you can see it regularly. Every time you do, ask the Lord to help you believe it. Pray that He will help you to see yourself the way He does. Give Him praise when He does.

Week 13 Day 6 | *Names for You: Masterpiece*

When my wife was pregnant with each of our children, we played it "old school" by waiting to learn the gender. There are so few guaranteed good surprises in life, we thought we would have fun, knowing we would be happy no matter what. Of course, that presented some logistical issues.

You can imagine how hard it was deciding what colors to use in their rooms. Registering for baby clothes. Listening to "guaranteed" gender predictions. Having to repeatedly justify to others our decision to hold off finding out. At times, it was almost as if we had offended them by waiting! The biggest issue was, of course, the names.

Society insists that parents must come up with at least one set of first and middle names for both genders. Sometimes more, just "in case."

Well, when each of the children were born, we were prepared. They were named Jordan, Myla, Genevieve Grace ("Gigi" for short), and Silas.

Now what's interesting is that—whether you learn their genders early or not—they grow into their names. They start behaving and looking like their name is perfect for them.

Jordan seems like a Jordan. Myla acts like a Myla. Gigi and Silas's names fit them as well, both in appearance and personality. Whatever their name, it's an unmistakable part of their personality, written on their ancestral DNA for the rest of their lives.

Our names are a part of our identities. They help define us. They're engrained in who we are. It's pretty rare to wake up one day and feel like our names don't fit us anymore.

I've never gotten out of bed and said, "Wow, something feels off. You know, I don't think my name works for me anymore. I don't feel like 'a Matthew.' From hence point forward, I shall be called Ted!"

Today is a *big* day—Day 90! The final day of this particular journey in fitness and spiritual accountability. Regardless of the physical results you've seen, my hope and prayer is this:

You've been encouraged.

You've developed a more intimate relationship with the Holy Spirit.

You've grown in your understanding of God's love for you.

When we see ourselves through God's eyes, we can't help but to experience growth.

We need to allow His names for us to be written on our spiritual DNA, and to adopt them as our own.

Once we believe what He says about us, we don't suddenly stop seeing ourselves that way. Not when we really believe it to be true.

Unfortunately, we're out of days to expound upon their implications for your fitness and your entire life.

Studying the many names God attributes to us is amazing. When we read them in succession, His regard for us is overwhelming.

A glimpse of the deep, astounding, and profound love God has for you can empower you to have victory in all things, your fitness included.

Take a moment to shut your door. Turn off the TV. Put your phone in another room. Find some solitude. I'm being serious. Take 20 seconds to get completely alone.

Now, silence the distractions. Prepare your heart and mind for the most remarkable, unique, and only pure love ever known . . . God's love for you.

Pray that the Holy Spirit would strengthen you. Pray also that He would help you believe what you're getting ready to read, even though it is undeniable truth.

As you read each name aloud, pause and reflect, marveling at the implications this has for your life.

This is you!

(OUT LOUD) Because of Christ and in Christ…

I am the **temple of the Holy Spirit** (1 Corinthians 3:16).

I am **God's worker, His field,** and **His building** (1 Corinthians 3:9).

I am **saved** (Titus 3:5) and I am **set apart** (Acts 26:18).

I am **holy** (Colossians 1:22) and I am a **saint** (1 Corinthians 1:2).

I am the **salt of the earth** and the **light of the world** (Matthew 5:13–14).

I am **called** (Ephesians 4), I am **complete** (Colossians 2:10), and I am **Christ's friend** (John 15:15).

I am **justified** (Ephesians 2) and I am **redeemed** (1 Corinthians 6:20).

I am **righteous** (Romans 5:19) and the **righteousness of God** (2 Corinthians 5:21).

I am **alive with Christ** (Colossians 2:13) and I am the **aroma of Christ** (2 Corinthians 2:15).

I am **purchased** (Ephesians 1:14) and **reconciled** (2 Corinthians 5:18).

I am **chosen** (Colossians 3:12) and **adopted** (Romans 8:15) and **part of God's family** (Ephesians 2:19).

I am His **ambassador** (2 Corinthians 5:20) and I am His **heir** (Romans 8:17 Galatians 3:29).

I am **accepted** (Romans 15:7), **forgiven** (Romans 5:1) and **free** (Romans 8:1).

I am **loved** (Ephesians 3:18–19). I am **wanted** (Romans 5:8).

I am **very good** (Genesis 1:31).

I am a **new creation** (2 Corinthians 5:17).

I am … His **masterpiece:**

"For we are God's masterpiece. He has created us anew in Christ Jesus, so we can do the good things he planned for us long ago."–Ephesians 2:10 (NLT)

In Christ Jesus, we are God's finest work. No matter what has happened in the past 90 days, or what will happen in the next 90, we are God's masterpiece. Because of that, we can do the good things He planned for us long ago.

Prayer

Father, thank You for seeing me through these 90 days. Will You forgive me when I ever take for granted how wide, how long, how high, and how deep Your love is for me? Please help me keep You as the focus of my life's ambition by relying on your Holy Spirit to power me—day by day, one step at a time. Amen.

Meditation

You are the Master and I am your masterpiece.

Daily Spiritual Exercise

Ephesians 2:10 says that we are God's masterpiece. Get out a sheet of paper and write down, "Because of Christ Jesus, I am God's masterpiece." Next to it, write down the implications this has in your life—what it will enable you to accomplish, how it affects your struggles, how it equips you for victory.

Then, post it somewhere you can see it regularly. Every time you do, ask the Lord to help you believe it. Pray that He will help you to see yourself the way He does. Give Him praise when He does.

I Have a Favor to Ask

You did it! I am so proud of you. I am hopeful you've been blessed by our adventure together. I prayed that your relationship with the Lord would deepen and that He would empower you to bring Him glory with your mind, body and spirit.

If you would like additional support or would like to go through the devotional in community, I believe you'll find being a BodyTithe.com member invaluable. BodyTithe.com is your "gym" in between your workouts. The tools, content, and resources available exclusively to members will motivate you, enlighten you, and give you confidence as you navigate what God-honoring fitness looks like. You'll be strengthened and encouraged as you are surrounded by like-minded Jesus followers seeking to bring glory to their Creator.

I'd also suggest you check out my Faith-Powered Fitness podcast. It's a free resource available through all the top platforms (Apple Podcast, Google Podcast, Stitcher, TuneIn, and Spotify). Each episode is educational, engaging, and edifying. After listening, you can't help but to feel both encouraged in your fitness but also in your heart, mind, and soul.

As I mentioned in the *Introduction*, there is a **free** "Leader's Guide" available for you to walk others through the 13 weeks of material (visit www.bodytithe.com/leadersguide). After downloading the guide, you can simply copy and paste the daily updates into a group on social media like Facebook, a message board forum, in text or emails, you name it. The Leader's Guide explains the process in detail, minimizing the burden on the leader. Will you prayerfully consider leading a group? Not only will you be a blessing to others, you might be surprised at how God blesses your own journey for a second time.

I am praying for many more to win spiritual victories—regardless of their physical results—through the message and lessons in *The Body Tithe*. **With that in mind, I have a favor to ask.**

Would you please take a moment to write a review of *The Body Tithe Devotional* and post it on Amazon.com (or wherever you purchased your copy)? The review doesn't have to be long or fancy, just a few short sentences of how the book helped you and/or what you learned from your 13-week journey.

The quantity of book reviews can be the difference between reaching a thousand people or a hundred thousand. Sharing how *The Body Tithe Devotional* impacted your fitness and your relationship with our heavenly Father might help more lives be changed.

Thank you again for going on this journey with me. I know your time is valuable. I trust you found the daily readings to be spiritually refreshing and life-giving encounters with our God who loves us beyond measure.

Remember always that what He requires, He provides. By the Holy Spirit in you, you are thoroughly equipped to honor Him in everything you do . . . your fitness included!